Ants in my Brain

A daughter's brain injury survival
story – a mother's perspective

By

Sally-Ann Mowbray

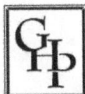

**Grosvenor House
Publishing Limited**

This book is published by
Grosvenor House Publishing Ltd
Link House
140 The Broadway, Tolworth, Surrey, KT6 7HT.
www.grosvenorhousepublishing.co.uk

A CIP record for this book
is available from the British Library

ISBN 978-1-83615-189-0
eBook ISBN 978-1-83615-205-7

"Hope" is the thing with feathers
That perches in the soul
And sings the tune without the words
And never stops – at all

EMILY DICKINSON

Contents

P... is for positivity

E... is for embrace

Foreword

by Dr Colette Griffin MBBS MD FRCP
Consultant Neurologist

I am honoured to write the foreword to this book. I am also honoured to have played a very small part in Rosie's journey. As a doctor, there are always patients whose stories live with you for many years after you have cared for them. This can be for many reasons. Rosie's is certainly one of those cases.

Our paths first crossed the morning of the accident. I could not get to work as the road was closed, and the other route to work was packed with traffic. As I tried to find a route with moving traffic, little did I know at the time that it was Rosie who had been injured.

I took over Rosie's care as soon as she was stepped down from the neuro-intensive care unit. Rosie was very critically injured, and very agitated. She required 1:1 nursing and intensive therapy input. It was very unclear to me during that first meeting with Rosie what the future held for her.

Rosie was deeply in post-traumatic amnesia, but I was struck by a feeling that underneath that she was very graceful, strong and driven. The other thing that struck me immediately was the wonderful loving family who were with Rosie constantly. Her parents and siblings were always serene and kind, which given the internal devastation they must have been feeling, took great inner strength and courage. They were all always involved in her care, learning about neuro-rehabilitation and actively helping Rosie along the path at every stage.

The road where Rosie sustained her injuries was on my route to work each day. As I passed by each morning and each evening, I would sit in traffic and ponder the fact that tomorrow is never a given for any of us. I would try to imagine what lay ahead for this beautiful, driven young woman, and what path her life would take going forwards.

This book is a wonderfully written insight into the world of traumatic brain injury from the point of view of the family and friends of a major trauma patient. It is very hard to read at times. I do hope it will help all those families who find themselves treading the same path. In those first few hours, days and weeks, I cannot begin to imagine the fear and uncertainty that loved ones and patients go through. The more information that patients, their families and friends can access the better. I do hope that reading this book will help those patients and families realise that hope, determination and love will always win the day.

I was delighted to bump into Rosie in the supermarket recently when I popped out of my clinic to get lunch. I could not have been more delighted to hear about her life and her next great adventures. As we both parted ways I felt a huge surge of pride, amazement and wonder at the power of the human body, mind and spirit. There may have been a tear in my eye.

The thing that still stays with me to this day a decade later, is the man who was on his way to work when he saw Rosie lying in the road. Without hesitation, he lay down on that cold road, covered Rosie with his coat and

Introduction

I am going to take you, from my perspective as a mother, on the journey of my daughter Rosie's recovery from serious acquired brain injury. It's a true-life story of hope. I ask you to bear with me, as I am not a writer; but what I hope to do is to offer you insight into how a traumatic brain injury can impact the life of a loved one and how this can affect the wider family.

One particular reason why our family's story may also be helpful to others is that Rosie did not follow any predictable pattern of recovery. But every brain is different. We were told and read what to expect at the various stages and how to understand the scales and charts that track progression and outcome; but there were months without any sign of a response, even though Rosie was awake and moving her body. We were hungry to learn stories about other brain injury survivors that would encourage us and increase our knowledge but there seems little out there and, with most articles having been written in America, we found few that related to our own situation here in the UK. My book is based on a simple, practical daily diary that I kept while Rosie was in hospital; and I talk to her at regular interludes throughout the book.

Being a private family, we find ourselves feeling quite exposed and often, it seems, analysed by professionals and many others, which isn't easy. So why am I prolonging this by writing a book? The simple answer is that if our story can give hope and courage to brain injury survivors and their families experiencing similar situations to ourselves, if it can enlighten others and lead them to a greater understanding about this silent disability and to think twice about protecting vulnerable heads, it will all be worthwhile.

By writing my practical and often light-hearted account, I would like to be able to connect with families and many others on an uncomplicated level. I wish to encourage others to have the strength to keep positive during the long haul of recovery and, when facing the worst, to hold on to the hope that our brains have amazing powers to heal, even though circumstances look very grim for many months and sometimes years. I speak from my heart as a mother.

~

Rosie's journey started at the side of the Durnsford Road in South London, then continued to the major London trauma hospital of St George's in Tooting, followed by her transfer to The Wolfson Neurorehabilitation Centre, firstly at St George's and then at Queen Mary's Hospital in Roehampton and, after discharge, to the family home in Dorset for community rehabilitation and beyond.

Rosie's father Adrian and I have now been married for over thirty years and have four adult children who live and work in and around London. Adrian manages a caravan park in Dorset where we have lived for the past twenty years. Our children are our world, the most important and treasured people that we are so thankful and privileged to have in our lives.

Our family had a life change in 2001 when the farm Adrian managed in Devon had a Foot-and-Mouth disease outbreak. Adrian was made redundant, we lost our home, and we also had to cope with a family bereavement during this difficult time. I wrote a daily diary then, which was published and is now an enduring record of that period of our lives, and which helped us all to come to terms with those events. Through that challenging time with our young family, we built stoical resilience; and I am convinced that this helped us all cope with the extra-large curveball that has been thrown our way.

౷

I dedicate this book to my daughter Rosie, whose steely determination, strength of character and positive spirit have inspired me to write, with her permission, about her life-changing story. I also dedicate this book to my other children, Edward, Pollyanna and William, whose coping mechanisms, strength and support have been truly remarkable throughout. To Adrian, my soulmate, my rock, and my constant. Last, and by no means least, to all brain injury survivors the world over – you are amazing humans!

Rosie is the second of our four children. Here is a brief summary of her life up to the point of her accident. Growing up, she was always a lively, happy child with a strong will. Living on a farm gave our children the freedom to explore the world around them, to use their imaginations unbarred and to have the space and freedom to develop themselves as individuals. We have always been grateful for that.

Rosie left The Woodroffe School in Lyme Regis at the age of sixteen to study childcare at the local college. She would catch the bus at 7am to take the ninety-minute coastal journey to Weymouth, returning at 7pm, and never missing a day, even when she was poorly or through bad weather – a work ethic she has strongly maintained throughout her life so far.

After a couple of years, she decided childcare wasn't really something she wanted to pursue as a career. With working life now beckoning she decided to chance her luck; and, arming herself with a bundle of her CVs, she distributed them to as many fashion retail outlets on the high street in Exeter as she could, in the hope of securing work of some sort. She was duly rewarded with a weekly eight-hour shift split over two days, managing a clothing concession at Topshop.

So then began her life of taking the bus into Exeter – another hour and a half journey – to complete these shifts, barely breaking even financially but always hoping, if she proved herself, that she might be given more hours in order to increase her experience within the fashion industry. This indeed happened; and after eighteen months of full-time employment she decided to try for a place at The London College of Fashion to study for a degree in Fashion Management.

Having left school without the qualifications she needed, she applied to do a one-year access course to enable her to progress to undergraduate status. I clearly remember the day we went up to London for her interview. It was early January; the snow had been falling relentlessly all night. We suggested to her that we call to rearrange, but Rosie was in total disagreement; so, after preparing ourselves with shovels, sand, warm clothes, food and a thermos we set off from Dorset to John lay talking to her and comforting her. In a world where we may sometimes worry about the future of both humankind and this wonderful earth we live on, that single act of kindness, the love of Rosie's family, and the sheer strength and determination of the human spirit as evidenced by Rosie, are all true wonders to behold.

I hope you find this book informative, enjoyable and a great read. I certainly did.

Dr Colette Griffin

H... is for healing

November 2014 – January 2015

Chapter 1

From Roadside to Resuscitation

10 November 2014

Text: Hey Mum, have booked my train to Cambridge for Wednesday 12th :) Looking forward to seeing you and having a nice day shopping. Will text you when I arrive. Love you lots, Rosie xxx

Text: Hi love. Excellent. See you there and have a safe journey. Love you lots too xxx

Adrian and I are going to Cambridge tomorrow for a few days to attend a work conference and I am meeting Rosie, who has taken the day off work for a bit of retail therapy and lunch on Wednesday and perhaps a bit of Christmas shopping too. RIGHT: have I sorted everything? Cases packed and ready – tick. Fizz and glasses – tick. Dog sorted – tick. Cat sorted – tick. Toenails painted – tick. As I lie in our bed that night, I touch its wooden side as I have done on so many occasions before. Touching wood that all the children are safely home from wherever they have been.

With the younger two in the last years at university and the older two having finished and starting out on their careers, it feels as though Adrian and I are both about to embrace the next stage of our lives. It feels good to have nearly broken the back of the university years and maybe it is time for me to think about my next chapter now that the children have all fled our nest and are forging their own paths in life. Yeah, we have cracked it; and now it's time for us to think about our own future plans. Time out in Myrtle, our 1972 much-loved bay camper van; holidays perhaps; visits to old friends; visits to the children and no more grubby student floors to sleep on and endless, exhausting trips to move offspring in and out of halls and houses. Time to contemplate our years ticking down to retirement, maybe. I muse on the shape of things to come as I fall gently into a restful night's sleep... But life doesn't always leave you alone like that...

11 November 2014 – Remembrance Day

7.30am: *Arrgghh!* Who is ringing me this early? Thought I would be woken as planned with Adrian bringing me my wake-up cuppa! Half awake, I view the number. I don't recognise you, so sod off and give me a few more precious moments of sleep...

BANG! That thud of Adrian's hand on our wooden bedroom door will resonate in my head for years and come back to catch me out when I least expect it, always evoking clear memories of this day and what it came to mean, the moment our lives were stopped in their tracks. That's what trauma can do when it makes its bed in the hippocampus of your brain.

Adrian has answered the call meant for me. "Lal, we need to get to London now!" he yells, his voice resounding with a panicky sharpness, a tone I have not heard before. "Rosanna has been involved in an accident and I have the Metropolitan Police on the phone. They have asked me if we are anywhere near Wimbledon and that they really didn't like relaying this news over the phone but she has been hit by a car and sustained pelvic, leg and chest injuries while she was out running at silly o'clock this morning; and, as we are in Dorset, they are trying to arrange a police escort for us." He stands stunned, almost unable to take on board what he has just said to me.

I'm not sure what happens the moment information like this is given to you. I guess at the time these are just words that don't quite make sense, sentences that seem out of the context of our normal everyday conversation. Right now, as I am writing this some years later, feelings of sickness and dizziness flood over me. I remember getting up out of bed and into overdrive, on auto pilot, in a matter of seconds. Rushing frantically from the bedroom in a frenzy of panic, getting into the shower, putting shampoo, conditioner and shower gel on somewhere, not in the right order or in the right place. Not sure if I even washed it all off or out. I needed time to think but I had to think quickly.

We call each of the other children in turn to tell them what's happened, a very painful thing to have to do at long distance as we know they will be distraught receiving this news. We know nothing other than what the police have briefly told Adrian. Our children's silence reflects the shock they feel.

Adrian wonders if, after we have seen Rosie at the hospital, we should go on to the work conference as planned . "No, I don't think it's like that," I say; and we both realise quickly that we are entering into unknown territory. Adrian heads up to his office to cancel his place at the conference and informs the caravan park staff what's happened. He sorts care for Monty our dog. Monty had been coming with us and we were due to meet Edd, our eldest, halfway so that he could look after Monty for these few days. I grab a few bits of clothing and we get into the car and leave.

This November day is dull and grey. The rain is streaming down on the windscreen as we drive to London, our minds full of questions, our emotions keeping time with the constant metronome of the windscreen wipers, keeping time with our thoughts and somehow stopping them from getting out of hand. During our journey, we have various calls from the police in charge and they decide that as we are making good progress, it is quicker for us to carry on driving on our own than for them to organise a complicated escort transfer through each county. They advise us of the severity of Rosie's injuries: on a scale of 1 to 10, these are about a seven. I think they left the worst bit for the hospital staff to tell us when we arrived, being conscious of the fact that we were travelling as fast as we could on a very wet day.

Radio Two reminds us of the day and time. Normally on Remembrance Day as the 11am two-minute silence approaches, we all stop respectfully to remember those whose lives were stolen through war and then carry on our days as normal. Today, Adrian and I sit in almost unbroken silence throughout our journey.

We have been informed that Rosie is in St George's Hospital in Tooting, a major London trauma centre. We have been instructed to make our way to the resuscitation unit which is situated in Accident and

Emergency. We understand that Rosie's flatmate Lauren has been first at the hospital, having made her way there immediately once she received a call from Rosie's sister, Pollyanna, and is waiting for us to arrive. Pollyanna has called me too to say that she could not settle in her lectures so is on her way to the hospital from her university in Winchester.

After negotiating the heavy London traffic, we eventually find a parking slot in a side road some distance from the hospital. We walk fast around the perimeter pathway of this huge and unfamiliar setting, searching for the A and E department, missing it completely and having to backtrack. Eventually finding it, our hearts drop as the queue is long, stretching out onto the pathway. We innocently join the back of it and seconds later a staff member spots us and beckons us forward through the doors towards two police officers. We experience a few black looks from some people waiting; I'm sure they felt we were being rude by jumping the queue.

We are desperate for the loo so are given the directions to make ourselves comfortable. Looking back now, I reflect that ignorance is bliss: we just had no concept of the enormity and seriousness of what was about to come our way – which, at that moment, was probably a good thing.

Where are you? and what have you done? What are we to expect when we see you? Can I hold you and comfort you? Or is this all out of our control, something bigger than anything we have experienced before...

We are ushered into the relatives' room accompanied by a staff member and the police officers who hand us a small plastic bag containing Rosie's house keys and her mobile phone.

We then experience every parent's second worst nightmare. Two doctors enter the room and proceed to tell us in the simplest way possible the extent of Rosie's injuries. "I shall start from the head and work down to the toes," said one.

We brace ourselves for what's to come. "Your daughter has sustained a serious brain injury and this is by far the worst of her injuries. Rosie is on a scale – she may never wake up, she could make a full recovery or she may fall somewhere along this scale. She has been put into a medically induced coma. She has multiple skull and facial fractures, a broken shoulder blade, broken ribs, a punctured right lung, pelvic injuries and broken tibia and fibula and her ankle has been displaced; and I don't expect you to have retained any of that."

I'm not really sure how anyone begins to digest this information; but as for not retaining any of it, that certainly did not happen to either of us. We retained every single bloody bit of it but had no real idea what it all meant.

We proceed into the resuscitation room to see our daughter. As we walk in I see Lauren, Rosie's flatmate, her face ashen and tense, and I immediately go to give this very brave young woman a 'mother hug'. She wobbles and a nurse finds her a chair to sit on. She tells us that she had been asked to identify Rosie but can only really do that from the pile of torn and bloodstained running clothes situated on the floor beside her bed.

As I turn to the bed I find it difficult to connect my daughter with the person lying here in front of me. Yes, she is my daughter, but not the vivacious, vibrant, lovable character that we know so well. Her head and body are so swollen it's hard to see where her neck meets her torso. Her hair, drawn back from her face, is crusted with dried blood; the large gash on her forehead is stitched up. Her badly bruised eyes are swollen and closed, her face unrecognisable. Her body is covered with nicks and scrapes and bits of tarmac from the road. Countless items of equipment surround her body and her right leg is in a brace. She is still. The only thing that's intact – bizarrely – is her toenail varnish, which is typical of her.

As we take a moment to digest this shocking scene, I turn and see that Adrian is on his knees. I bend down and help him up as we are being asked to accompany Rosie as she is transported through the hospital to the neuro intensive therapy unit on Atkinson Morley wing.

We move swiftly though the hospital corridors, the staff carrying the equipment that is keeping Rosie alive, and the three of us following behind in anxious silence. Passing through the double doors and into the Intensive Therapy Unit (ITU), Rosie's bed is wheeled to an empty slot near the end of the ward, and the staff busily link her up to the multiple monitoring and drug-dispensing equipment stands that surround her bed. She has a ventilator to do her breathing for her and a line of five or six life-saving drugs administered directly into her jugular vein to keep her alive and her vital organs stable. I try to keep focus on what is happening to Rosie, but I quietly fear we must be in the most critical of places within the hospital.

Before we arrived, Rosie had a number of CT scans to enable the staff to ascertain the extent of the damage to her brain as well as assessing the possibility of further bleeding and damage occurring.

The ITU resembles Star Trek's Starship Enterprise control room which, on reflection, is pretty much what our brains are to us all: our own unique Starship Enterprises. There are twenty or more beds lining two sides of a large room with a dominant control centre in the middle. Each bed has a pedestal at the end of it from which members of staff continually monitor changes in their patients, the most critical having twenty-four hour, one-to-one observational and medical care. The lights and bleeps are continuous. After being given a run-through of the expected hygiene routines – hand cleanser before and after entering the unit and fresh plastic aprons each time we are by the bedside – we are given chairs to sit on as we try to acclimatise to this alien environment which we anticipate will become Rosie's home and ours for some time to come. Pollyanna has now joined us; she feels sick and faint at the sight of her sister. It's hard to bear, as a mother, seeing your children like this when there is nothing you can do other than comfort.

Over the course of the day various members of staff come over and introduce themselves and, with the police, try to help us create a picture of exactly what happened this morning.

Apparently, Rosie had been knocked down at a pedestrian crossing while making her way across the road at about 6.15am during her 'before work run'. A kind and helpful gentleman on his routine journey to work heard the impact, witnessed Rosie flying through the air and went to her aid. He called the emergency services. Then covering her motionless body with his coat to keep her warm, he proceeded to lie down beside her, talking to her continuously in the hope that this would keep her brain from shutting down. In retrospect, this was crucial in keeping her alive; and this selfless act of human kindness is something we will never forget. We are forever indebted to him for his brave actions on this day.

When the police arrived, they observed the road users driving thoughtlessly around Rosie in order to continue their morning journeys, almost oblivious of her and the gentleman helping. They immediately rerouted the traffic to protect Rosie and themselves. One policeman who aided the medical team held her broken leg straight while the medical team applied a leg brace. He said it felt like holding a bag full of pasta.

The Helicopter Emergency Medical Service (HEMS) was on the scene within minutes and inserted a chest drain at the roadside since Rosie's right lung had collapsed. With no response from her and with a Glasgow Coma Scale of 5 that was sliding rapidly downwards, they immediately put her into a medically induced coma. Her leg was stabilised and, as the early morning traffic was still light, she was transported by road to St George's Hospital.

Later that afternoon, we take a much-needed break from Rosie's bedside in the relatives' day room that's next to the unit and have our first cup of tea of the day. We had had no time to think about eating or drinking anything before we left home this morning and, as the day has unfolded, this seems to have come last on the list of priorities. We have no appetite. The four of us sit silently, numb with shock. As we sit in this communal room with other equally anxious folk, an elderly mother enters, crying and shaking her head at her family who are all eagerly waiting for news; and this is swiftly followed by an intense wailing and outpouring of grief. We then observe many members of the devastated family streaming into the unit and surrounding the bed of their loved one who has sadly just passed away. These faces reveal the depth of their grief and pain; and this family now begin the long bereavement process, a sequence of events the likes of which we desperately hope will not come our way too. However, this gives us an indication of the variety of situations we will come to accept as normal over the coming weeks.

Pollyanna and Lauren encourage Adrian and me to take a much-needed breather in the hospital grounds. We walk the corridors and stairs, through the hustle and bustle of hospital life, and once outside we take a few steps and a few deep breaths but remain silent for most of the time.

We arrive back to find that Pollyanna and Lauren have moved to a smaller family room within the ITU as the shocking scene in the day room had been too much for them. Will, our youngest, has now joined us and he too struggles to comprehend what's happened. It is here that we are met by an experienced neurology doctor and given our first introduction to brain injury. He explains that at this stage it is impossible to assess Rosie properly as she is in a coma and they are trying to stabilise her. Over the coming hours, days and weeks we may start to be able to build a picture of how her injury may have affected her, and her potential outcomes.

During our discussions, Lauren asks if Rosie might still die. The doctor tells us then that the first seventy-two hours are critical and, at this moment in time, the answer is yes, she could.

Later in the evening, we all leave the hospital when the unit closes to relatives for an hour, enabling the staff to attend to their patients before the last visiting session of the day commences. Rosie is now stable but unresponsive so we will go back later for the last visiting hour in the hope that her condition will have improved.

We arrive at Merton Road to the flat Rosie and Lauren share. It is such a strange feeling to be here without her. Rosie and Lauren had been firm friends through university and lived together during their final year. They decided, after leaving their student life behind, to set up a home together now that they have both become working professionals; and they have been happily living in their new flat in Southfields for the past two and a half months. These two peas in a pod are real creatures of habit, little home birds.

This morning when Rosie didn't return from her run, Lauren sent a text to her to ask where she was; and receiving no reply, she decided to call the police to report a missing person, thinking Rosie might have been abducted. She was told they could hardly put out a "missing person" alarm for someone who had been absent for just fifteen minutes. Little did she know about the scene that was unfolding barely half a mile up the road as she started making her way to work.

We lightly joke at this recounting of Lauren's story and imagine that before long Rosie will be strutting out of the hospital wondering what all the fuss was about. She certainly has the strength of character, but I think even this will be a test for her. A test bigger than anything she has experienced in her life before.

The *Evening Standard* and the Wimbledon paper report that Rosie had been knocked down by a lorry, which was not true; but what they do report correctly is that she is fighting for her life. We find this disturbing to read; and absorbing everything that has happened today is immensely difficult.

After feebly attempting to eat our supper and failing miserably, Adrian and I return to the hospital to find the unit a little calmer but still filled with some of the grieving relatives from the family who had earlier suffered a loss. We want nothing more than to be with Rosie. Her body feels so lifeless, so cold; she's pale and still. I want to hug her close to me but am scared to disturb the equipment that surrounds her. This all seems very unnatural.

This place of despair that surrounds you… You are so cold. I gently snuggle the worn, cellular hospital blankets around your hands and feet to warm them up but it has no effect; it's as if your limbs have died already. You are eerily still, so unlike you. If only you could wake up and see this; but then again, that might be far more painful for all of us to bear just now if you did, my love.

Before we leave, we are approached by the senior doctor who we saw earlier. He reassures us that we need to look after ourselves, eat and rest, since we will need all the strength we have for the days and weeks ahead. It's not an instinctive reaction to have when your daughter is the one who is suffering; but as we come to realise over the course of time, his words were vitally important to take heed of. We have to keep our energy tanks filled in order to keep strong and positive for Rosie and the other members of our family.

We arrive back at the flat and go into Rosie's room for the night. We see her things just as she left them this morning: work clothes neatly on her bed ready to be changed into after her run, her train tickets to Cambridge for tomorrow on the chest of drawers; and I swallow hard as we retire to her bed.

Our sleep is restless and broken. We wake at various points in the night and sit almost bolt upright in shock. We have visions of her body being tossed through the air like a rag doll – visions which are difficult to 'unsee'. The saying 'your blood runs cold' has never been so apt: this sensation of ice-cold blood pumping speedily from my heart around my shell-shocked body is now a familiar feeling, the adrenaline rush forcing me into reality. This happens time and time again for weeks to come.

Chapter 2
Critical but Stable

The following morning Adrian gets up and makes us both a cup of tea. We sit silently in bed staring blankly at the cracks in the bedroom wall, our internal dialogue a mismatch of muddled questions and angst. We occasionally pass our thoughts to each other but don't really come to any conclusions, shock still getting the better of us.

We head to the hospital and take up camp in the day room alongside the many relatives and friends of other patients on the unit. We all take turns in our bedside vigil as only two persons per patient are allowed at any one time. All of Rosie's closest friends are privately informed and we make the decision not to announce any information on social media, watching her account like hawks in case anything unnecessary is posted. This decision, although not right for every family, feels appropriate for us.

Rosie is critical but stable; and that's all we can expect at this stage.

During the day, the staff try to reduce her sedation a little to see if they can get any response. They try unusual ways to achieve this, loudly shouting her name into her ear. I can still draw the sound to my mind of the clinical nurse specialist shouting "ROSIE!" into her ears. They pinch into her collar bone in the hope of getting her to flinch, dig a pencil very hard into her cuticles, asking her to do the 'thumbs up' and demanding that she squeeze their hand hard – only to be met with a blank-eyed, squinted stare and stillness every time. Initially, this makes for very uncomfortable viewing but soon we find ourselves regularly carrying out these exercises on her, ever hopeful of a sign of reaction.

The staff perform another CT scan which thankfully reveals no further bleeding on her brain. We are given the information that every brain injury is different and that, even though some scans may show up a lot of damage, the outcomes may be better than predicted. Conversely, other scans may reveal minimal damage, and the outcomes may prove much worse. This aids our understanding a little and we begin to realise what an unpredictable injury this is for the medical profession as well as for the patient and their family.

During the afternoon vigil, we notice Rosie make a slight arm movement and attempts to lift her eyelid; she also gives a little cough. It is amazing how these simple and basic reflex signs of life start to give us hope.

Rosie now has a nasogastric feeding tube (NG tube) inserted through her nose and down into her stomach. This will keep her almost continuously fed with the right balance of chemical food to keep her alive, and her dietitian monitors this closely. Rosie has always taken good care with her diet, being almost too healthy sometimes; but this has contributed to her good general health and physical condition and, we hope, her recovery too. It's quite difficult to see her now with her body being pumped full of this alien substance. Its light brown, liquid consistency resembles something that might be found in a chemistry laboratory or even put into a car's engine.

We are informed that an intracranial pressure monitoring bolt (ICPB) has been inserted into Rosie's skull to measure her brain pressure which is constantly fluctuating. In a young person, the brain normally fills the skull cavity so there is little space for a swelling brain to go. This vital piece of monitoring equipment can only be in place for about a week, which is a relief since it plays havoc with our emotions and is hard to ignore with its high-pitched bleep every time her brain pressure gets high or she shows signs of stress. It looks odd to see her with this contraption protruding from her skull – not quite the 'must have' hair accessory of the moment, that's for sure.

The staff move Rosie to the opposite side of the unit. The windows are larger on this side and give us a feeling of lightness as we can see the setting sun from here. Days afterwards, we are told that this side is for the more critical patients. As we reluctantly leave her bedside for the night, we reassure ourselves that she is still alive and stable for the moment, and for that reason we must keep hope.

ॐ

Rosie's older brother Edd arrives today and as we sit by her bedside for ten minutes or so in shocked silence, I see his face drain of colour; and so we retreat to the day room to recuperate. I can't imagine what it must feel like for the other children to see one of their siblings in this state.

This environment is so alien to us all. It's a massive sensory overload mixed with indescribable emotional pain and shock. It's almost dreamlike at times, as it's hard to connect our daily reality with what we are all experiencing now.

Over the next couple of days Rosie develops pneumonia. Apparently, this is relatively common and most patients have this at least once during their stay on this unit; and she is treated speedily with antibiotics.

The process of lungs being suctioned is one of the most unbearable sights to witness, especially when it is happening to one of your own; and it is one I hope I never have to see again. The suction tube is inserted into Rosie's lungs through her ventilator and this triggers her limp and frail body into a jerky, rhythmic spasm of coughing as the infected secretions are extracted, and she coughs as if in the most unimaginable pain. This must be done regularly to lessen the infection but it is tricky, as she is still on a ventilator.

The pot that collects these secretions could put you off your lunch forever. I turn to the next bed and see a mother whose son is going through the same process. She can't bear to watch, either, and turns away, choking back her tears.

I stand by and watch as this process is performed on you, my love, time and time again; it never gets any easier. I wonder just how much pain you can feel. Your expression indicates that it hurts you so much. Those clean and heathy lungs that have served you so well are having to cope with so much; they will have to prove themselves now, that's for sure.

As Rosie is given her second blood transfusion, we sit beside her bed and observe little movements again: a very slight turn of her head, an eye half open; and we imagine that maybe she can hear our voices as we talk closely to her, holding and stroking her arms and hands. We are fooled into thinking she is squeezing our hands in response to our command, but sadly this is not the case. It's a little bit like seeing your baby smile for the first time, only to be told it's just wind.

Towards the end of the first week, we settle into a daily routine centred around our visits to the ITU which start at 10am and finish at around 7pm. Occasionally we return at 8pm if we feel so desperate and in need of seeing Rosie for reassurance before we go to bed ourselves, or if she is showing signs of instability again. We are still in limbo as these critical first few days could so easily go one way or the other.

By now Dani and Greg, the partners of Edd and Pollyanna, have visited and have been through the same initial shock of seeing Rosie. We take refuge daily in local coffee shops in Tooting and Colliers Wood. We share our feelings with each other as much as we can articulate them right now. Just having a brief change from our hospital surroundings and finding something comforting to eat and drink really helps to keep us all going, giving us short interludes from the relentless emotional angst we experience from hour to hour and day to day.

For Adrian and me to have our other offspring and their partners around us gives us the strength we need to carry on each day. They all have busy lives and we are all juggling. They take a break to buy us some much-needed underwear as the few bits of clothing I bundled hurriedly into a bag on Tuesday morning are running out and essential additions are very much needed. On their return, the family produce a set of mugs to use in the day room for our endless rounds of tea and coffee – mugs with the abbreviations OXO, LOL and OMG printed on their sides in large letters, the family's way of lifting the spirits and keeping us all going. We see the irony and laugh, wondering what the other day room visitors make of this.

That evening, as we drive away from the hospital, Adrian and I decide we must make plans for the forthcoming days and weeks as much as we can. We pull up on the roadside opposite the flat and sit quietly and with some degree of despair, trying to work out a solution as to how we go forward from here. Adrian's job is a caravan park manager and we live and work in the Dorset countryside. Thankfully, the park is closed to the public at the moment so, apart from winter maintenance, it's a relatively quiet time of year. It seems a million miles away in contrast to the scenario we have been thrust into here in London. In order to keep his job and to keep our income, we plan for him to go home tomorrow, Sunday, to organise work for the staff for the coming week. I, thankfully, have stopped work for a break so am able to devote my time to Rosie. We need to create a balanced routine now as the way things are looking, we are going to be here for some time to come.

That Sunday night I climb into Rosie's bed alone for the first time in London.

I find your pyjamas under your pillow and pull them close; your smell is on them. I imagine they are you and hug them to me. My body is overwhelmed with emotion and sadness for you and I weep and sob with every fibre of my being until I ache all over. My love, what has happened to you? Please don't leave us. You are so strong; please fight though your weakness and be brave. I will wait until you come back to me. I am here.

I wake the following morning exhausted from restless sleep but the release of emotion has helped me and I sob and sob until I am all cried out.

Pollyanna arrives at the flat and she too has had a night similar to mine and we both feel as if some pain has been lifted, as if we are both a little lighter. We make our way by bus to the hospital to start this second week. Rosie's team of highly specialised neuro-physiotherapists ('physios') have been working hard to create casts for Rosie's left foot to stop it drooping and setting in one place. This needs to be done regularly and in stages to bring her feet back to the right angles. Her right leg is still in its brace awaiting an operation and will have the same procedure once it's mended. We sit beside Rosie, holding and gently stroking her hands and talking to her: "Who is going to win *X Factor?*" and "Who's in the line-up for *I'm a celebrity... Get me out of here!*"; the weather conditions, our dog Monty – anything that comes into our minds. We intersperse this with sitting silently, observing and patiently waiting.

Adrian returns from Dorset this Monday afternoon and recounts his last twenty-four hours to me. Driving away from St George's Hospital, going 150 miles in the opposite direction knowing that all he wanted to do was to be by Rosie's side, had been very hard. Sometimes, you feel so helpless being by her side but even more helpless when you are not.

It had been a struggle for him to say goodbye to us all; phoning his mother and shedding some tears was a release for him. He arrived home in the dark to a cold and empty house but with a warm welcome from Monty and set about his chores. He sorted post, put our dirty laundry on to wash, and dried it ready to bring back upon his return journey, and planned work for the next week. As he was going about the kitchen he came across my teacup and teapot still sitting next to the kettle on the worktop, as it had been since we left so hurriedly. He had to swallow hard to hold back the ever-threatening tears and continue, starkly reminded of that frenzied Tuesday morning when our lives took a different turn to the one we had planned.

Shortly after his return home, the house is filled, firstly with a dear friend bringing a hot stew for his supper; and then other friends follow, bearing food for him to take back to London for us all. These friends are devastated by what's happened to Rosie. Many of their children have grown up with ours and they cannot comprehend what this must be like for our family, and they want to help in some way.

When Adrian returns home to Dorset each Sunday night after this first visit, the house soon fills with friends armed with boxes and baskets of food, parcels and treats for him to bring back up to London the following day. This happens for some weeks and we all look forward with eager anticipation to what delights will lift our spirits each day for supper. Many a homemade Dorset cake has been appreciated while we are sitting in the day room and on the corridor seats of St George's. These extremely kind gestures, these treats of lovely homemade food make all the difference, especially when the last thing you feel like doing at the end of these emotionally exhausting days is cooking.

We have to make a plan for the care of Monty for the longer term and, although he is getting much attention and walks from our friends who live locally, we need to make sure he is happy and safe and not adding to our current worries. Edd and Dani offer to look after him in Hertfordshire for the foreseeable future where he will have plenty of space to run and lots of affection. Adrian and Edd agree a suitable meeting place on the M25 to transfer him over.

Edd, being a bit further away from the hospital, sometimes feels a bit helpless, so it helps to keep his spirits lifted now that he feels he can do something useful to help. Monty is much-loved and, as we have no idea how long we will be away from home, it is reassuring for us all to know he is safe and that we can nip up and visit him from time to time.

Chapter 3

Waiting for the Storm to Pass

Over the next couple of days, the staff try to reduce Rosie's sedation again to see if any responses occur. She is starting to take over a little more of her own breathing, so they are hopeful about starting the ventilator weaning fairly soon. As they start the sedation reduction, we observe Rosie's arms and legs making alarming, involuntary movements which I can only describe as disturbingly disabled in their look. Her limbs start to flail about, and her feet and hands tense up in a display of rigid, extending movements; she sweats profusely and gets very agitated, which in turn sets off all her monitors. The process we are told is called 'storming'. No one can really give us much information about this disturbing process other than that it happens when people possibly suffer from more serious and deeper brain damage. This information brings us down to earth with a sobering thud and we fear so much for her now. These storming episodes can be managed with drugs and generally pass in time. I guess right now we are literally 'waiting for the storm to pass'.

When you know nothing at all about brain injury, you fear the very worst in everything you witness. Storming, particularly, is something that is very hard to imagine and desperately hard to watch, and we search Google (never a good thing) in the hope that we may find out some more information; but there isn't really anything out there that gives any definitive answer.

The staff are concerned at Rosie's very odd limb movements but to us at times they are quite typical of her. She is very tall and gangly and flails her arms and legs particularly when she runs, so sometimes it's hard to differentiate between normal movements and something more sinister. We feel a bit silly when we mention this to the staff and perhaps we are trying to kid ourselves into thinking things are better than they are, although I'm sure a person's natural bodily movements have to be taken into consideration.

Adrian and I need to take a breather away from Rosie's bedside as these episodes of storming are difficult to watch for any length of time. We decide to pick up a sandwich from the food store in the grounds of the hospital and head down to a little park in Colliers Wood. The day is bright, and the late autumn sun is shining. As we walk up Blackshaw Road, discussing the events of this morning, an overwhelming sense of anger and frustration flood over me. I kick the nearest tree I come to, stubbing my toe in the process. These trees are big and old and shouldn't really be messed with or treated like this, but it makes me feel so much better to release this tension that has been building up inside me. Whenever I have returned to this road and passed that tree, I have said a slightly humble 'sorry' to it and a 'thank you' for being there. We enter the park in Colliers Wood and find an empty bench amid the huge, winter-prepped trees and sit in a state of numbness and confusion, trying desperately to imagine what the future will hold for us all. We arrive at the conclusion that we must just try as much as we can to take each day as it comes and to hold on to as much hope as the staff can offer us at any given time.

It has now been seven days since her accident and the intercranial pressure bolt has been removed from Rosie's skull. It's a relief to see this and to see that the lovely nurses have washed all evidence of dried blood from her blonde hair and created two long plaits. It gives us a real lift in spirits to see something more normal happening to Rosie, something that has personalised her.

The staff who care for her here at St George's are amazing. Everyone seems to have found a soft spot for Rosie and are rooting for her to recover and make progress as much as we are. They take time to support us as a family, too, and this helps to alleviate our worries to some degree.

Over the next days, Rosie's dreadful storming episodes become a little less frequent and have also subsided in their intensity. The staff have managed them carefully and she is responding to the medication. She seems more comfortable now. Her eyes are beginning to open a little more and she makes an attempt to grab at her ventilation tube. Apparently this is a very normal reaction and we are told that this may indicate the start to her becoming aware, although more often than not it seems she is just catching her long fingers in the tube as she involuntarily gesticulates with her arms from time to time.

Today the maxillofacial (max fax) team come to take impressions of her mouth and jaw in preparation for the long and painstaking operation to rebuild her broken face. Her upper jaw has been pushed back significantly over her lower jaw and she has six loose teeth that are completely separate from the rest in her upper jaw. Her face looks completely flat on one side but her skin is unbroken, for which we are thankful. I suggest to them during our discussions that Rosie has always been slightly dissatisfied with her nose so I'm sure she would be grateful for a minor nose job, a "buy one get one free", perhaps, while in the process of her operation. We're not sure if they plan to put that on the list but we wait to see.

The surgeons ask us if we have any recent photos of Rosie to help give them an idea of her bone structure and facial features before her accident. We offer them one that was taken when she was last at home in Dorset a couple of weeks ago. How ironic that Adrian took such a good close-up of her so recently, as we sat by a glowing fire enjoying our gin and tonics and chatting.

I touch very briefly on that memory I have of you that weekend. We ran together on the local cliffs at Stonebarrow Hill, embracing life, the fresh air, the beautiful scenery. Exactly how are we here now? In this mess, this confusion, this ugly scene of suffering. Is this a dream that we will all awake from shortly and go back to our daily lives? I hope so, my love, I really do hope so...

When Edd and Dani next visit again, they notice improvement, which is great for us to hear. For the family who see Rosie daily, it's difficult to have any real gauge of progress so those who know her so well and have short breaks between their visits really encourage us and bring

ANTS IN MY BRAIN

a breath of fresh air and energy to the days when we are flagging.

We regularly continue with the rounds of stimulation in the hope of a notable and consistent response but so far we have nothing tangible to report. We have a tendency to overdo the 'thumbs up' and the hand squeezing, in desperation at times, hoping for something, anything, that indicates Rosie is making progress of some sort. We regularly show her photos of herself with her friends, family and Monty to see if we can get any recognition. An old friend has sent her printed photos of the good times they spent together and her bed is now surrounded with little gifts and familiar objects in the hope that they trigger something within her. We spray a little of her familiar perfume, all in an attempt to jog her senses back into action.

There are now rumours that the staff may start weaning Rosie off her ventilator next week which is a positive sign, as this has been delayed a little due to her storming episodes. Her lungs seem to have picked up strength and we now have reinforced hope that she may be able to breathe on her own again. We keep our fingers tightly crossed.

Over coffee with Edd and Dani, I recount my fears to them surrounding Rosie's storming episodes and my concerns for the future. Edd offers solid words of comfort and positivity: "Mum, we haven't buckled when we have been faced with difficulties before and we are not going to buckle now;" and this gives me the courage I need to carry on. When Adrian is away from me, I vow to recount those words to myself when I next hit a low point. We decide to pop a photo of Rosie at her graduation ceremony in July by her bedside. The staff are amazed to see how beautiful she looked before her accident.

I sit alone on occasions by your bedside and look upon your graduation photo, those happy memories of your amazing achievement, all that hard work paying off to begin the next exciting step along your life's path. I glance back down to where you lie now, so sick and so frail, empty of everything you once were, my darling child. I can't do anything to make things better, to wipe away this helpless pain for you or for me or for any of us.

Pollyanna and I decide we need to start looking after Rosie's appearance and her personal care, since lying in a hospital bed day after day can cause such deterioration. She has started to lose weight and her skin has become increasingly dry and flaky. We start the week by calling into the shopping centre on the way to the hospital to pick up some toiletries: nail files, creams, soft flannels and soothing gels to massage into Rosie's hands and feet. We need to feel purposeful, so attending to her personal needs is therapeutic for us and, although she may not be aware of us doing this for her, it may bring comforting sensations to her body.

When we arrive, we set about our care plan and this brings a sense of calm and connection with Rosie that we desperately crave. The staff observe this and encourage us, giving us little hints and tips about the areas that are prone to deterioration and how to negotiate her tubes and lines. We have built up such a lovely rapport with some of the nurses. Many are around the same age as my own children and others are mothers like me and we chat about their lives and ours at brief opportunities during their demanding and lifesaving work. This helps to pass the time away.

The doctors carry out an EEG brain test today on Rosie. This test tracks and records brain activity. Small metal discs with tiny wires are placed onto the scalp and these send signals to a computer to be analysed. The doctors are relieved to find no evidence of fits and seizures and can report an amount of brain activity which is very hopeful.

The ITU environment is full of monotonous, stimulating sounds which make it hard for patients to get any sustained period of peaceful sleep. Over the last few days, we have noticed Rosie's closed eyelids flickering a lot in a pattern of REM sleep, so maybe this is due to the continuous broken sleep pattern that she has. She looks permanently tired and pale from this.

Rosie has improved enough for her ventilator to be removed completely today and, with the aid of an oxygen mask, she is beginning to breathe on her own. We are so happy for her and the relief for us all that progress is finally being made is incredible.

At the end of her two weeks since admission, Rosie has her two-and-a-half-hour leg operation and we are thankful her broken bones can now start to mend over the next ten weeks without bearing weight. Her pelvis has been x-rayed again and these fractures are now stable and will mend on their own, meaning that she may eventually be able to walk again, however unreal this prospect seems at the moment.

Sadly, she has to be put back on the ventilator briefly as she struggled to breathe during her operation; but she is now stable again and back to breathing on her own.

Adrian and I take a visit to see Rosie's work colleagues today in central London, walking through busy Piccadilly to Beak Street, unsure exactly as to where we are going but excited to meet her new work chums. She has only been working at this advertising company in a new graduate role for a few months but has made some lovely friends, who are keen to be updated on her progress and desperate for her to return. Rosie has a very infectious nature and a fun-loving spirit; they miss her a lot.

After our visit, we sit in a café having our lunchtime sandwich, the loud noise of music and chatter feeling so intrusive that we can barely hear each other talk. It feels very odd to be in the busyness of the West End and hard for us to connect our girl lying in St George's neuro intensive care unit, so fragile, with the office full of the vibrant young people we have just visited. We sit and wonder if she will ever be back there again but must, at least for the time being anyway, place these anxious thoughts at the back of our minds.

As Christmas is in the air, we decide to take in some familiar festive songs and play them to Rosie. Christmas has always been her favourite time of year and we are hopeful that the sounds may in some way stimulate her. We do this in short bursts as we are told overstimulation can lead to her brain shutting down.

In these early stages after injury, the brain can only absorb little bits of information at any one time, but it is sorely tempting to overdo this in our desire to see any reaction. This does promote some agitation and sweating from Rosie and we wonder if somewhere in this muddled brain of hers there has been a connection. I'm sure, though, if I were played 'I wish it could be Christmas every day' repeatedly, I too would break out in an agitated sweat.

Max fax advise us that all being well, Rosie will go down for her face operation tomorrow and – fingers crossed – we can put another tick in the box for operations; there's always a 'but'.

Chapter 4

Ups and Downs on ITU

I am woken with a jolt this morning and the dreaded 'no caller ID' is displayed on my phone. I instinctively know it's the hospital calling me and they advise us to come in as soon as we can.

Rosie has rapidly developed another chest infection and experienced breathing difficulties during the night; a blockage of mucus has led to her left lung collapsing. This is not good news as her right lung is still fragile and recovering after it had to be inflated at the roadside immediately after the accident. The staff have had to reventilate her and increase her sedation and she has been given her third blood transfusion.

Everyone on the unit is shocked at this and we sense that Rosie's recovery is less hopeful now. It may be that a degree of oxygen starvation has taken place, and this could be detrimental to her brain and increase the risk of further damage. Sadly, her face surgery has had to be postponed which is a real setback; and she is showing signs of another bout of pneumonia.

As we sit beside her bed digesting what has happened and being comforted by the staff, I feel a gentle touch on my shoulder and, as I turn and glance upwards through my tears, the lady doctor says softly, "But she is still breathing." This is a very hard sentence to hear when you are so desperate for more than just this; but in acute medical situations like these, I suppose it's the starting block the medics need to continue preserving life.

That evening, on recounting this downward turn to my dear friend who is fighting her own battle with terminal cancer, her comforting words to me were, "Where there's life, there is hope, darling." Bless her, she knows strength more than any of us; and I shall never forget her saying this as it encouraged me to continue and to face each day with optimism.

The following day the decision is made for a tracheotomy to be performed. This is a rather crude procedure that enables a patient to breathe through a tube inserted through an incision into their windpipe which is then linked up to a ventilator. With Rosie continually having infections and inconsistent breathing patterns, this is the right decision for her; and once her face operation is performed, her jaws will be wired together for some time afterwards, so it is highly likely she would need it anyway.

Once this tricky lifesaving procedure has been completed, she settles a little but seems to wince as if in pain. She is on continuous pain relief so this is increased accordingly. We are given advice that this will be a far rockier road than was previously thought given her lack of response and the medical and physical difficulties. Conversations about her ability to work or live independently again are difficult to have. I recall one afternoon when our youngest son Will was with me and a rather overzealous junior doctor quite inappropriately and blatantly telling us that, in his opinion, Rosie would not work again or live independently. Saying this as definitely as he did caused Will to almost collapse and the staff managed to get a chair for him just in time. After this news, we both sat down for some time by Rosie's bedside and wept, the pair of us together.

Later that same afternoon, Adrian and I are given a letter stating that Rosie is unable to manage her financial affairs, should we need this proof. We are advised that she may need to claim benefits in the longer term and suggestions of finding a good solicitor are put forward. We are all brought to a very low ebb indeed by this information and the implications it has for Rosie's future.

We take on board the advice that has been given to find a reputable solicitor who specialises in brain injury cases. Making a claim against the insurance company of the car driver is something that doesn't sit right with us morally; but after careful consideration and, under these circumstances, we feel we need to protect Rosie's future if possible. The police don't have enough evidence to bring court proceedings but emphatically suggest we make a civil claim.

We were fortunate (although at this moment that word in the broader sense could not be more inaccurate) that she hadn't just fallen down the stairs or had a naturally occurring acquired brain injury, for instance a stroke or brain haemorrhage. Under these circumstances, there would have been no insurance claim to pursue.

We set about finding a recommended solicitors' firm through the website of Headway, the brain injury association, and make an appointment to see one of the senior partners at their Richmond offices.

On arrival, Adrian and I are shown to a meeting room, given a cup of coffee and told that the solicitor will arrive shortly. We sit waiting, mulling over in our heads what questions we are likely to be asked.

I am glancing through this office window that overlooks Richmond Green and clock a large, familiar-looking ancient tree. My eyes fall beneath its boughs to the grassy picnic spot upon which we sat only months ago. You had eagerly waited all day at work, your advertising intern post in Richmond, to open your degree results and Dad, Pollyanna and I drove up from Dorset with a picnic to surprise you. We sat in the hazy sunlight of that warm June afternoon and toasted your achievement and shared your hopes and dreams on that day for the bright future that lay ahead of you. The total contrast in a matter of months to what we were doing then to what we are doing now is unbelievable in every way.

I am jolted out of my daydream as the solicitor enters the room and to the stark reality of some very difficult questioning. He asks, in the most sensitive way possible, these questions.

"Is your daughter doubly incontinent?"

"Can she breathe for herself?"

"Can she feed herself, walk, talk?"

The list is endless. And so we begin the start of another challenging journey that will run parallel with our daughter's brain injury recovery. Unbeknownst to us, this will be a very long and difficult legal journey.

Tooting is slowly becoming a familiar place for us all now and, although there are parts of London that Adrian and I know reasonably well, the only tentative association we both have with this area of the capital is through watching the 1970s sitcom *Citizen Smith*. It's strange to be using regularly the Tooting Broadway tube station that Wolfie Smith made so famous in this great comedy. I think we could benefit from his iconic fist pump, sending his 'POWER TO ROSIE!' energy up and over the rooftops and on to the intensive care unit of St George's and to Rosie to aid her recovery. It's a busy and bustling multicultural environment and, as we walk aimlessly through the streets to take our daily lunchtime breaks from the hospital, we are very aware of how many ambulance sirens regularly fill the air. As we are all still very emotionally raw, these sounds shock and penetrate our minds. We wonder if any of these ambulance crews went out to Rosie on the day of her accident, what it was like for her, and what kind of emergency they will have to deal with now.

We have now sourced the most comfortable coffee shops and have become some of their more frequent visitors. It's quite possible we sit alongside many others unaware that they could be distraught families just like ourselves. We begin to feel quite attached to our new environment in a rather strange way. Subconsciously, we now expect that Rosie will be here in St George's for some time and we want to draw stability and comfort from wherever we can.

It's the last weekend in November and all the family and Lauren are here in force. Generally, it's quiet on the ward during the weekends with temporary staff covering.

We all feel frustrated at the lack of progress but encouraged as we see Rosie a little more settled now with the ventilator removed from her 'trachi' (tracheotomy) and replaced with a smaller oxygen tube. Her lungs, although getting stronger, are still being suctioned regularly to remove stale and infected mucus as she can't move to stimulate the natural coughing process.

We all keep a wide berth when she coughs as we don't fancy being in the firing line of projectile mucus when it's coughed through her trachi opening. It can reach distances almost impossible to imagine with its jet-propelled force and we take bets as to where it may land next. Seeing the funny side helps us cope since observing is still so very painful; her whole body curls up in the most horrendous motion which leaves her incredibly exhausted. We begin to observe little changes. She blinks a little more and moves her arms around, which heartens us all.

The staff inform us that they intend to prop Rosie upright as a change of position could be good for her brain stimulation and they might, if that is successful, manoeuvre her into a hoist and sit her on the side of the bed. We all start to get quite excited to see what will happen. This proves to be a very long and slow process and requires at least four people to assist as she has no control over any aspect of her head or body. This simple action we all take for granted takes some doing and afterwards Rosie is exhausted with the movement and change of position.

When she is back in her horizontal position, she immediately shuts down and we leave her sleeping and calm in the afternoon.

As Adrian heads back to Dorset this Sunday and all the family members go their separate ways home, I go back to the flat and Lauren and I discuss the events so far. Lauren mentions that one of her and Rosie's favourite TV programmes is *24 hours in A&E*, a medical documentary programme set in St George's Hospital. Not being particularly familiar with hospital programmes, I hadn't heard of this until now. Bizarrely, only a few weeks ago, Rosie had said to Lauren, "How odd would it be to watch this programme if you had been on it and could look down on yourself lying in a hospital bed!" If only she knew.

For Lauren, all she wants is for her flatmate to come back and life to continue as before. She didn't sign up for living with Rosie's parents; this is such a difficult time for us all and I try my hardest to be of comfort to her whenever I can.

As I crawl into bed and have my private sob again, I realise that tomorrow is December 1st. Christmas is looming and rather than lifting the spirits as it usually does, I feel a lead weight in my heart at the very thought.

Mondays are always a bit strange without Adrian, but Pollyanna and I have slotted into a regular routine now. Pollyanna is in her final year at university, trying to balance her dissertation preparations with daily visits to the hospital. She is incredibly strong and resilient, a great comfort to me; but I worry that this is going to have a devastating effect on all her hard work – and on Will's, who is in his second year.

I encourage them both, and Lauren too, to return to their respective daily work routines as much as possible. Rosie would be so upset if she felt her accident had stopped them from continuing with their work and failing to get their degrees. We can only hope she will be able to attend their graduations over the next two years, as they did hers just a few months ago.

During this next week, the physiotherapists manage to progress a little and regularly repeat the procedure of putting Rosie into a hoist. Her ever-diminishing, slumped body resembles that of a very elderly frail person, so it is quite a challenge. There is talk of putting her in a chair over the next few days to see if this can encourage any coordination control or response, as her chest infections are improving and she seems a little more stable than previously. The movement of getting from bed to chair via a hoist can be a very demanding one. Her head and body have no control at all and this often leaves her very sleepy, but it is progress of a fashion and it's good to see her body in a different position and out of bed even though it is just for very short bursts at a time.

Chapter 5
The Possible Paths of Recovery

Later in the week, Rosie's neuro physio coordinator gives us some basic information about the Glasgow Coma Scale (GCS) which measures a patient's level of consciousness after an injury. As the patient improves, they are assessed using the Westmead Scale, a scale which measures the length of Post Traumatic Amnesia (PTA), a state of confusion that happens after a brain injury. The length of time a patient is in PTA can generally indicate the severity of their injury; and these are the points below that we are given. It is well worth remembering that this is a guide and every brain is unique and the responses and outcomes vary immensely:

Severity of Injury	Length of PTA
Very mild	Up to 5 minutes
Mild	5–60 minutes
Moderate	1–24 hours
Severe	1–7 days
Very severe	1–4 weeks
Extremely severe	Over 4 weeks

Given Rosie's lack of response and with no real starting point or benchmark for assessment, we are told that as well as sustaining three haemorrhages to her frontal lobes, it's possible she has sustained a 'diffuse axonal' injury. This injury sends the brain into a ricocheting motion on impact, twisting within the skull and causing many neurons to sever in the process, thus causing more generalised brain damage. This injury doesn't show up on brain scans, so it is difficult to gauge the extent of the damage that's occurred. The impact of this damage will only really come to light in time, if and when she recovers.

We are slowly and succinctly talked through the two possible pathways for her recovery. Firstly, if Rosie continues to stay in this minimal conscious state for any considerable length of time, she would be transferred to the Royal Hospital for Neuro Disabilities in Putney for longer term in-patient care. The second option, if she wakes up and becomes responsive again, would be to transfer her to the acute ward on the third floor of the hospital. Once she has transitioned through the Post Traumatic Amnesia stage, she would go to the Wolfson neuro rehabilitation centre based at St George's to continue her recovery.

We hope and pray it's the second of these two scenarios. We are put in touch with the South West London office of Headway, the brain injury association, and given booklets from St George's to educate ourselves about brain injury. Within the booklets we find some useful information for families affected by brain injury and the five different stages of emotional reaction that are likely to occur:

- Shock, panic, denial: "Please let him live."
- Relief, elation, denial: "He's going to be fine."
- Hope: "He's making progress, but it's slow."

- Realisation, anger, depression: "He's not getting back to his old self."
- Acceptance, recognition: "Our lives are different now."

Although sobering to read, this did help us to identify our own feelings to some extent and are pretty accurate reflections of a family's recovery process as time goes on. Acceptance is the hardest stage of all.

We are constantly thirsty for knowledge about what has happened to Rosie and our family consult Dr Google (again, never a good thing) for more information about Diffuse Axonal brain injury.

Big mistake! The outcomes are generally very poor for people who sustain an injury of this nature, and it makes very disturbing reading indeed. This news is quite shocking and not easy to grasp in one go.

I discover from the internet that Richard Hammond, the TV presenter, suffered a Diffuse Axonal injury when he sustained a brain injury in 2006. He regained consciousness fairly soon after his accident and has since made an amazing recovery. This gives us some hope, as the recovery statistics are quite devastatingly low. Will Rosie be lucky enough to be in that top few percent of survivors who make a good recovery?

As Adrian and I sit alone, digesting what's just been said to us, a sudden and quite intense feeling sweeps over me, almost a wave of connection within me to my daughter and a 'true grit' stoical determination that we are not going to give in to this information. Fooling ourselves? Maybe, but I know her; she is stronger than this; and this deep-rooted feeling, a mother's instinct, keeps me strong and positive. She will survive whatever the outcome. She is not going to be beaten.

I continue with my daily diary for her, little snippets of information that one day she may be able to read and so fill in the gaps of this missing period of time in her life.

I took a battering, but I've got thicker skin
and the best people I know
looking out for me.

'Get Better' – Frank Turner

Chapter 6

The Day Room

The ITU environment is steadily becoming a very familiar place for us all. After nearly five weeks, Rosie has been on the unit the longest since arriving. We see many comings and goings, both through death and progressing from the unit into life. Many patients are transferred to hospitals nearer their home to ease the financial and time burdens on their relatives.

When there is a death, the curtains close and the relatives surround the bed in these last precious moments that they have to be able to make memories. The body is then respectfully removed to make space for the next patient. I reflect that if there is anywhere where life and death are so basically inter-connected, it's here. Where there is life, we all cling to the positivity.

The day room is a small room directly outside the intensive care unit for all the relatives to take a breather from the bedside vigil. It changes from day to day, depending on the casualties who are admitted. The room has an array of mismatched chairs and a tall potted plant that sits next to a small window. When the space is free, we always make a beeline for the window area, as this pocket of natural daylight tends to lift our moods a little. There are basic tea- and coffee-making facilities and a small but adequate fridge in which to keep our communal milk and sustenance for the day. The toilet is adjacent to this room.

This toilet is my bolt hole that briefly holds me together. My moment to ground and get a grip. I need this space, even though it's time limited, so that I can walk back in and keep this pretence of control. You would understand this if you were my side of the fence, my love. I am bleeding inside for you, this unknowing, this tightrope we walk, inch by inch, daily. Waiting for something to happen for you – but what is next? I cannot go too deep into my thoughts for that.

Sometimes there is a sense of calm when we all sit together in silence, occasionally exchanging updates about our loved ones and our experiences of our time here so far. I remember so many times when relatives spoke of progress: "He's now doing the thumbs up" or "She's spoken for the first time" – feeling encouraged for them, but secretly saddened as still we have nothing to report. No sign of anything that indicates that Rosie is making the transition to consciousness.

On other occasions the whole room could be taken over by one family – sleeping bags, takeaway pizza wrappers, pushchairs and pillows. These are all signs of the instant upheaval and knock-on effects on the wider family when a traumatic incident happens to one of its members.

St George's sees people from all walks of life affected, as we are, by trauma. We sometimes see families and friends fill the day room with little awareness of, or empathy for, others around them. On these days, we set up camp on seats in the corridor nearby, as if needing to lick our own wounds in quiet contemplation. We are all thrust into this small space without warning or preparation and all of us need to be allowed to deal with our pain in the way that feels right for each one of us, and show tolerance towards each other's situations and beliefs as much as we are able.

The different ways we and our fellow inmates handle this alien environment is something we adjust to over the days and weeks and, in order to counteract the abnormality of this place we all find ourselves in, we have to lighten our load with a bit of humour. Sometimes this can be a bit dark but, as a family, we are always quick to see the funny and sometimes ironic side of life, even now. This may sound bizarre to some but it's definitely some sort of mechanism for coping and trying to remain positive under such testing circumstances.

We cheekily nickname the people around us. We have the lovely Mr Ponytail Man, Nicely Turned-out Lady, Bin Man and his brother, Motor Bike Man. Bin Man has been so-named because every time he lifts the dustbin lid to deposit something, he lets it bang back down with a loud, resounding crash. Our offspring decide to mimic this, much to our amusement, although always in an empty room so as not to offend. How I long for a 'soft closing' bin lid.

Some people fill the fridge with trays laden with posh food covered in large signs stating, 'Private food, do not eat'. It's very hard for us all to resist the temptation of sneaking a teeny-weeny bit of something delicious from their trays. This, and endless quantities of crosswords, codewords, word searches and sudoku help us all pass the long periods we spend cooped up in here.

Some relatives live quite a distance away from the hospital and the daily grind of travel adds to the burden of the situation they find themselves in. Headway and other brain injury charities can offer some financial support to families in our situation, but this can only be sustained for a short period of time. We all have this anxiety of not knowing and the future hangs over us all like a dark and gloomy raincloud.

We are fortunate to have Rosie's flat to provide a close-by roof over our heads and thankfully, Rosie is able to sustain the monthly rental costs for the immediate future at least. We would be extremely financially challenged if this wasn't the case, particularly as we have made the decision to keep Rosie in St George's for the consistency in her care. Our decision is based on the fact that she would be relocated to a specialised hospital in Southampton, more than two hours away from our home in Dorset, and we are sure this would complicate our lives even more.

As we enter the first weekend in December, we are encouraged to see Rosie move to the opposite side of the unit where two or three patients are monitored by one nurse. Surely this must mean she is starting to make improvement? She is becoming a little more awake but is still unable to hold her gaze on any one thing, even though her eyes are opening slightly more. Neither can she respond to any sort of command, despite us still continuing regularly with the now well-rehearsed loop of requests. Dani and Pollyanna open an advent calendar for her and repeatedly read her the cheesy daily quotes; not even this gets a response. It is, however, very encouraging to see the bedside area freeing up as she becomes less dependent on drugs and equipment.

Rosie is now being hoisted into a chair most days and she is managing to hold her head a little steadier with the aid of a neck cushion. We can now wheel her out through the double doors and into the corridor for very short bursts so that she can see the daylight through the large hospital windows that overlook Tooting.

The London early winter sunsets we see regularly from the unit are a sight to behold: beautiful, vibrant, autumn-coloured skies, which we want to magic inside to brighten this sterile environment.

I know you would appreciate these magnificent skies, the contrasting colours, the shadows and shapes, the twinkling of the stars peeping through, backdropping the rising moon. We used to sit outside so much during your childhood years, didn't we? Star-gazing, making shapes with the clouds – who would find the funniest face (usually Edd), and we would all laugh so much. Laughter is what we did together then; it feels we have to pause that sort of laughter for now.

Chapter 7

Dorset for a Day

This Sunday afternoon, after much persuasion, I decide to go home with Adrian to Dorset. Rosie is going to have her long-awaited face operation tomorrow so there will be nothing much I can do here other than wait around in the day room. As we will be back tomorrow afternoon when she returns to the unit, I feel it would be nice to go home even if it's just for a few short hours, a breather. This will be my first visit home since Rosie's admittance.

Driving away from the hospital fills me with tears of sorrow. Will she be okay? Are we past the living or dying phase? These questions and many more we mull over between us and the drive gives Adrian and me a chance to collect our thoughts and reflect upon what's happened since our lives were turned upside down. We shed tears and discuss the situation we are all in. It's strange how your lives can so swiftly transition from planning ahead with clear confidence to existing only from day to day. It's not until something completely out of the ordinary like this happens that you realise just how much the general consistency of life, the daily humdrum of routine is taken for granted. How I wish to have a slice of that in my life just now.

We arrive home to a place that feels a million miles away from everything. So much has happened in our lives in such a short space of time and my head feels very unsettled. I potter from room to room trying to adjust.

Making one cup of tea and sitting briefly, making another and standing, staring blindly out of the conservatory window into a garden of nothingness, my thoughts plunging to introspection and then back to that familiar feeling, that blank state of shock.

As I walk around the kitchen, I look up to my carefully strung bundles of onions hanging with pride on their hooks, just some of the produce from our ever-full veg patch. I squeeze them lightly to see how they are drying and find that each and every one has started to rot. How strange that this has happened during this difficult period of our lives. I don't want to think too hard about this.

I tentatively call the hospital to be told that the staff are washing Rosie's hair ready for her face operation tomorrow. I am warmly comforted by this thought and keep my fingers tightly crossed that we don't have a repeat of that previous November night before this operation was due to take place. She seems a little more stable now and less sickly, so I am keeping positive for her.

Friends pop around with the now regular welcome food parcels for us to take back to London and their hugs and kind words of encouragement cheer us both up. That evening Adrian and I sit by a warm and comforting fire in quiet reflection, bouncing off each other with our thoughts and our feelings. Surely, we have got to be luckier than this? But why? We are no different to any other family faced with such adversity. Why should we be luckier or unluckier?

Later, when we surrender to our exhaustion, we fall into our bed, Adrian not alone for this Sunday night at least and me, even if just for one imaginary moment, writing a different storyline of events from the last time I slept here.

When we return to St George's late the following afternoon, we walk towards the bed where we last left Rosie only to find another patient in her place. We are instantly informed that she has moved back to the opposite, more dependant side of the unit. Our hearts sink slightly, and we walk, with some degree of urgency, up the rows of beds looking for her. We come to a lady with blonde hair and a swollen face and seem to think in our muddled heads that this is Rosie. A member of staff, noticing our confusion, steers us in the right direction. It's crazy how your mind can play tricks on you when you don't quite know what you are looking for or what to expect.

When we come to Rosie, her closed eyes and her face are black and swollen with bruising, she has stitched wounds around her eyes and in her hair line indicating the points of incision, and she is sadly back to being ventilated through her 'trachi'. This immediately brings back to us the desperately traumatic images of the first day we saw her in the A and E resuscitation room. Her teeth have been solidly wired together to keep her jaws stable and these wires are barely visible beneath her bulgy lips. This implementation will enable the healing to take place without movement and sadly, she is back to being more drug dependant. The 'max fax' team arrive at her bedside and declare to us that the four-and-a-half-hour operation had been a success considering that they had been faced with, in their words, a 'box of cornflakes'. These surgeons are incredible. They have plated, pinned and reconstructed the whole right-hand side of Rosie's face, stabilising her jaws and loose teeth and repairing the bridge of her nose and both her eye sockets, all with very minimal external evidence. They give us the news that her teeth wires must be *in situ* for at least four weeks. This disheartens us somewhat and we so hope this does not hamper any progress Rosie may make, but we realise this will give the best chance for her face to repair to as near normal as possible. She is heavily sedated again for her pain.

Dad takes his first picture of you today since your accident. He hasn't been able to steel himself to do it before now and probably doesn't want this image to sit too close in his phone photo stream to the last one he took of you at home; that pain would be too great. He knows just how inquisitive you are as a person. From that day when, from your baby carrier on my back, you peered intently over my shoulder to watch me assist the ewe as she gave birth to her lamb, to your endless what, why, when, who and how streams of questions as a youngster, your lively mind never rested; and if one day you wake up, we know you would want to see this. It may aid your understanding a little of this surreal time you are unknowingly passing through.

The following day the staff remove Rosie's ventilator and she is breathing again by herself with a little oxygen to assist. She seems in considerable discomfort and thrashes her head around from side to side in what looks like continuous frustration. We sit and comfort her as much as possible and wonder if she is vaguely aware of the restriction now placed on her mouth. Rosie has always been a constant chatterer, the one who would be sent out of the classroom for talking during the lesson at school, the one who would brighten up someone's day with a witty comment or funny story. Perhaps, in her deep subconscious, she may be protesting about this restraint. How we wish she could communicate with us and tell us how she feels.

Over the next few days, as Rosie's pain relief keeps her stable, she continues to thrash her head from side to side in marked frustration. When they wash her hair, the lovely nurses caring for her notice a matted mass of hair at the back of her head, which has formed as she constantly turns her head on the pillow.

Pollyanna and I decide that we should start removing this chunk of hair. We nip up to Tooting and purchase every conceivable brush, comb and hair conditioner we think would be useful and try, together with the nurses, to tease the lump out. Rosie protests about this by forcefully pulling her head away from our hands, her agitation clearly evident through her gestures. Each day after this, and when she permits us, we try to free this stubborn mass from her hair, but it proves really tricky. Strangely it gives us and her nurses something constructive to do for her. It helps to pass the time, as we constantly invent new ideas to avoid our least favourite option – the dreaded scissors.

We still continue daily with our now well-rehearsed exercises and routines trying to get a response from Rosie, but to no avail. At times it feels like we have such an uphill struggle, but we must keep going in the hope of a breakthrough of some sort. We are encouraged when a loud bang happens right next to her bed and she wakes with a start, as this gives us hope that she can still hear.

Why do I revert to the baby years when I talk to you? It's as if we are starting all over again. Mummy, Daddy, Zanny ... Daddy, Zanny, Mummy. "Shut up!" I hear you say in my head, and I hear your siblings say it too. "You have always talked to us in an adult way, even when we were kids. Talk as you normally do to me. I am not the child you think I am; I am still me, the adult."

It's a week after her face operation and Rosie is having more periods of wakefulness than we have seen before. She moves her arms and legs about with a little more control and all the family members who don't visit daily are really encouraged by seeing this progress. They even feel she is sensing our voices now, although it would be good to have more evidence of this.

We have regular chats with the staff on the unit and they encourage us to start looking at Rosie's progress on a weekly rather than a daily basis. This was useful advice to hear and we plan to put it into practice as best we can. We realise we have subconsciously transitioned from moment to moment, worrying as to whether she will survive or not to something that has a little more permanence. This could mean the beginning of leaving the tentative 'life versus death' stage behind us, although it may be an indication that progress will be very slow from now on.

The physios continue their painstaking work, changing and altering the casts on Rosie's feet in order to bring them to right angles again. Little by little, improvements are made so that, if and when she can walk, her feet are not stuck rigid and on tiptoe.

We still can't really visualise Rosie walking again at the moment as she seems so far from this, but the experienced staff here understand brain injury and physical recovery at a far higher level than we do. Witnessing these regular procedures certainly gives us the snippets of encouragement we are looking for to keep positive. They certainly haven't given up hope for her and we remain loyally alongside them all, absorbing, listening and educating ourselves as much as we can.

Chapter 8
From ITU to Brodie Ward

The following Monday, we are told that Rosie will now be able to transfer from the ITU to a high dependency unit within the Atkinson Morley wing. We are extremely encouraged by this news after nearly six long and tense weeks in intensive care.

When Pollyanna and I arrive this morning, we find Rosie has been moved to a quieter side room in preparation for this.

As we sit by her bedside waiting for her to be moved, we notice a distinct change in her awareness. It's subtle but marked. She seems more active and attempts to launch her body into a sitting position but promptly flops back down with no strength or brain ability to keep upright. She then, slowly but purposefully, moves her left index finger to her head and lightly scratches her scalp. We can hardly believe we are seeing this movement, the first positive indication that her brain has function to coordinate a bodily sensation with a reflex action.

We are both ecstatic to see this breakthrough and a bit tearful too and can't wait to tell the family. Her neurosurgeon comes in to see us before Rosie leaves the unit and is very encouraged to hear about our observations. He confidently gives us hope that we should start seeing more progress of this nature over the weeks and months to come.

We accompany Rosie as the hospital porters transport her and her bed through the corridors of Atkinson Morley Wing and onto Brodie Ward. She is now resident on a four-bed bay in a much quieter environment. Her bed is positioned by the window, bright and airy, and it feels more like a general hospital ward.

As it seems much quieter here, we hope that Rosie will start to acquire more of a night and day pattern. I arrange with a nurse to help wash her hair the following morning and, as we do this, I take the decision to cut out the large lump of matted hair we have tried so earnestly to free without success. This is not an easy decision to make but we all hope it will grow quickly and, because it is near the nape of her neck, it is not really visible.

During my haphazard hairdressing session, the nurses appear from ITU to visit Rosie in her new surroundings and are extremely relieved that I have concluded that this task is now our only option as all others have been exhausted. They all miss her on their ward, just as we miss them. It felt safe having her there – not that she isn't safe here, but staff are thinner on the ground and have a wide variety of patients with more diverse needs to care for. Rosie had become one of their longest-staying patients on intensive care and one they showed great affection for; and I'm sure they want to keep track of her progress.

As Rosie settles into her new surroundings and the staff become more familiar with her jaw wires and tracheotomy care, we continue with the daily routine of commands, but this gets more challenging and frustrating as we are unrewarded every time. We show her photos and think that, in her calmer moments, she is holding her gaze on them a little longer. But it's as if she has a spell over her that's showing no real sign of breaking.

The change of environment seems to have caused her to become much more active and fidgety, pulling her body towards each side of the bed in a repetitive motion. She uses the bed sides as a grip to heave herself into a continuous, almost obsessive pattern from side to side that can last for hours at a time. This continues day after day and is very difficult to watch. At other, calmer moments, she just stares blankly for long periods at the padded bed side protectors that are designed for children's beds. These have animated pictures of elephants, lions and giraffes on them, so maybe it's the bright colours and simple shapes that draw her eyes, her re-emerging brain entering the start of a second childhood phase. This transient pattern of focus and sleep and periods of wakefulness bear many striking similarities to the patterns of new-born babies. Their tiny developing brains form as the pathways connect as they grow. It's just the lack of any liveliness that is so different in our current situation, and the absence of crying. Having had four children in the space of five years, I have had my fair share of crying babies, so I am relieved about this.

Rosie's work friends can at last send her flowers, a huge bouquet themed with Christmas-coloured sprays of every description. They are placed on the reception desk that sits just outside her bed bay for everyone to appreciate except her.

We start to increase the variety of interactions and try to engage Rosie in a few small clips of her favourite episodes of *Friends* to see if she can focus for longer periods. More Christmas tunes are played and their repetition, we hope, may stimulate her awareness; but nothing generates any consistent attention or recognition.

We still visit every day and for most of each day. Even though the visiting hours are a little more controlled here, the staff seem to turn a bit of a blind eye to us huddling continuously around Rosie's bed. We can't seem to alter this pattern formed in ITU and certainly don't want to miss any progress she may make, as it's become like a drug of desire and need for us all.

After a week on this ward Rosie develops a very nasty stomach bug. She is now looking quite emaciated, gaunt and weakened by this, and her weight loss has increased dramatically.

The nurses here encounter a real problem in replacing her catheter. After two and a half exasperating hours of trying she is taken back briefly to the intensive care unit for it to be done by more experienced staff.

As I carry out my daily massaging of creams into her now skeletal feet and hands, I ponder the question as to how this poorly bony body can survive in this state. Our bodies are quite remarkable as regards the limits they can tolerate and survive; her body is a far cry from the healthy and fit one that entered this hospital in November.

I feel such sadness and pain inside me when I scan your weakened and tragic body. I am tormented by your quiet mind, your vacant expression, those stone-hard staring eyes I long to penetrate to the person that I once knew. I hate this for you, my love, so much – this sickly, sad and sorry state that you are in. I am helpless in my desire to make this better: isn't that what mothers do, make everything better? I cry so hard for you, cry that you will recover from this and show us that you are you again, and only housed temporarily in a broken body and mind.

This is the week leading up to Christmas and I find myself becoming more and more emotional as Rosie is in such a poor physical state and still showing no sign of awareness.

As we walk around the seasonally decorated shops, pumping out the same old Christmas songs on repeat, we try to get some inspiration for the festivities and draw blanks regularly as to what presents to buy the family, our enthusiasm at its lowest ebb. We are acutely aware that this Christmas will be very different from anything we have ever experienced before.

Normally at this time I would have lists upon lists of things for us to do. For me: busily preparing and cooking the food for the big day, wrapping gifts, sending cards, choosing and decorating the Christmas tree, filling the house with an abundance of holly and ivy. For Adrian: perfecting his home-produced ham and making sure we have enough booze and chopped wood for some good fires as he shuts off from work for this much-anticipated two-week break, whilst we await our offspring and their partners' homecoming at various times to celebrate together. We all look forward to the traditional family Christmas we have had for the past twenty-seven years. During the time when we lived and worked on a farm when the children were much younger, we made our own entertainments a lot of the time, as there were always animals to feed and jobs to do on Christmas morning. We lived quite remotely and didn't have other family particularly close, so we made our own fun and amusements centred around our life as it was then. The board games and charades have long since remained an integral part of our festive rituals to this day. This year, I have to console myself by reminding myself that this is just one Christmas; and next year may be different again still.

Before Adrian returns to Dorset for the last time before work shuts down for Christmas, we decide to cheer ourselves up as much as we can over Sunday lunch at a local pub with Pollyanna and Greg. We still need to take some respite regularly from the clinical surroundings of St George's to recharge our batteries. It feels quite disconcerting to sit surrounded by many others so jovial with Christmas spirit, happily chatting about their plans together as the holiday season approaches. This just underlines again to us all how distant we are from any sense of what normally happens for us at this time of year.

Just as we are about to finish our lunch, my phone rings with no caller ID. The hospital are calling to inform me that Rosie has had to be admitted back onto the Intensive Care Unit. She has been urging to vomit due to her stomach bug and, as the staff on the ward she is on are not adequately trained in using the emergency teeth wire cutters – which might need to be used if she starts to choke – she has been readmitted as a precaution.

We arrive in haste back at the intensive care unit; its familiar friendly faces are there to greet us. It feels comforting to know Rosie is so well looked after, and the staff reassure us that she is here just as a precaution and will return to Brodie Ward when they feel sure she is out of danger. They have put her in a large pair of baggy green hospital pyjamas, not the most attractive we have seen but they do make her look a stone or so heavier at least. It is a nice change from the standard blue and white gown we have grown so accustomed to seeing her in since her admission many weeks ago. Rosie makes a reaching gesture towards me which is encouraging, and her eyes seem to focus periodically on the lights of the Christmas tree that's now on this unit.

After twenty-four hours of observation on intensive care, the staff feel she is settled enough and safe to go back to Brodie Ward. Sadly, another patient has taken her bed spot in this short space of time so we must wait for another bed to become free. As she still has her 'trachi' in place, she can only go back to this small, high dependency side ward where there are trained staff to care for her.

After a brief and anxious few hours overnight in Dorset, Adrian returns to the hospital just after the staff and I move Rosie back to Brodie Ward. We spend a little time this afternoon making her surroundings comfortable, adding a few Christmas touches. I think the short stay back in intensive care has settled her stomach and she seems a bit more awake and a little less sickly.

I observe her making a brief swallow and she closes her lips at the same time. This voluntary series of reflex actions is something the staff have been very keen to see happen for some time. It's a marked step forward, as it possibly indicates that Rosie's brain stem may be less affected than we all think. It could indicate the possibility of her eating food again, of talking and breathing independently. Not that we can get too carried away by these prospects just now. These little signs I note in my daily diary and they prove useful 'bites' of observation for the medical teams and give us, as a family, a benchmark of weekly progress, which is encouraging.

In preparation for the Christmas period and the ward staffing plan, Rosie's bed is moved closer to the staff station to help make observation easier. Her chest is also giving her problems again so needs to be kept a close eye on. The increase of spasticity in which her muscles continuously contract and stiffen, which is a condition related to her brain injury, make it challenging for the physiotherapists to negotiate around. She has suddenly become increasingly more active, thrashing her limbs around more frequently but with no control at all. This makes it problematic for the staff to keep her (and themselves) safe as she now has more solid casts on her legs, to help repair the breaks, and on her feet, to prevent them from drooping. When she thrashes about, those long limbs flail and wallop whatever happens to be in their path and we all experience, at some point, the sheer force of them; and it hurts. After spotting Rosie on the floor one afternoon, sitting almost in the prayer position at the foot of the bed, the staff endeavour to search the hospital for a longer bed to try and contain her, and this helps to some degree.

We have a long discussion with Rosie's neuro physio coordinator, who has become a lynchpin for us throughout our time so far at St George's. She advises us that Rosie is possibly entering a phase of Post Traumatic Amnesia. This is a transitional period in which patients can display some alarming and often erratic forms of behaviour. However, this process is the gateway for the start of recovery and the beginning of a person's ability to regain some function. If this happens for Rosie, the medical teams may be able to pinpoint in more detail her damaged areas. We are extremely encouraged by this news, the one and only Christmas present we could wish for this year, and we eagerly wait to see what happens next.

Following our discussion, and in line with the advice given to us, Rosie starts to become increasingly agitated. She pulls more frequently at the lines that feed drugs into her arms and tries to pull off the oxygen tube that's linked up to her trachi. This causes concern as, if she manages to ease out the tracheal tube, she will compromise her ability to breathe in a big way. She periodically scratches at a small scar on her face as if it's irritating her, perhaps indicating that her facial wounds are repairing well. The max fax team review their work and are pleased with the healing progress so far. The next step will be to wean her off her tracheotomy if she is able, but this will have to wait till the New Year, after her teeth wires have been removed. This is frustrating as progress is slow, but they can't afford to risk this removal process with a closed, wired-up mouth.

Chapter 9

Christmas of a Different Sort

Christmas Eve is now upon us and we keep calm and busy washing Rosie's hair and painting her toenails before the 'big day', stimulating her at brief periods with photos of her work colleagues in their Christmas jumpers and reading out heartfelt messages from them and other friends. I wonder if she will ever remember or recognise any of them again.

'Twas the night before Christmas and all through the house, not a creature was stirring, not even a mouse' ... Our dusty, old and tattered copy of this much-loved Christmas Eve favourite is still sitting somewhere on the bookshelves at home, waiting to be read to future grandchildren. My favourite bit when you were younger, and Dad and I were permanently exhausted, was 'and Ma in her kerchief and I in my cap, had just settled our brains for a long winter's nap'. I longed for moments of peace and quiet; the idea to 'settle one's brain' for a long stretch sounded like heaven then. I have rewritten this passage for this year's Christmas Eve... I yearn for your brain to unsettle, my love, to wake up, to be lively and active just like it used to be. I can't help but wonder if you will ever come to remember this book or our Christmases of the past?

The family encourage Edd and Dani to take their biannual Christmas break in Sweden with Dani's family. Although they both leave with heavy hearts, it's imperative we try to carry on with normality as much as we can in order to preserve our mental and physical wellbeing. Will and Pollyanna will be with us and we plan to 'make the best of it'.

Over the past weeks, we have settled into a routine at the flat, enhancing things to look a little festive despite our current mood. Lauren, Pollyanna and Will have decorated a cheap and cheerful Christmas tree and hung up an array of Christmas cards containing warm, personal messages of support and hope for the coming year.

Life has to take a shape of some sort – nothing like normal but a shape, nevertheless. We all put on brave faces and plan tomorrow, even though Christmas is the last thing we feel like celebrating. We have a luxury Christmas hamper kindly donated to us by a friend containing everything for lunch, thus relieving any pressure from cooking as our main chunk of the day will be visiting Rosie. I have often thought these hampers an extravagant and rather lazy option for Christmas lunch; but after seeing just how many people use this service for one reason or another, ourselves now included, I have become far less judgemental.

It's a very strange feeling today, this Christmas Day. Normally our family would wake up and open our stockings together, have a nice breakfast and walk down to the sea at Charmouth to watch the brave Christmas Day swimmers, in a variety of entertaining costumes, run into the freezing water (and out again, pretty quickly).

We would then return home for present-opening around the Christmas tree and enjoy a large festive lunch with lots of laughter, cocktails, board games, quizzes and charades into the late evening hours as the fire embers fade. I think now of our family home miles away in Dorset – empty, lifeless and cold – and glance over at my younger two, sitting on the sofa together, their solemn faces expressing exactly what we are all feeling. Again, I remind myself that this is just one Christmas, and just how fortunate we are under normal circumstances to have the family Christmases we do. There is nothing like the London streets, particularly at this time of year, to reinforce and remind ourselves never to take what we have for granted.

We head over to St George's after breakfast and are quite taken aback by the number of visitors it has on this day, giving us a strong feeling that we are not alone in our situation. We all congregate in the small day room on this ward, passing the time as best we can until we are called through to see our respective patients.

As we sit with another family, their lively little boy starts strumming on a small guitar he has been given as a Christmas present. We all find this amusing and it briefly offers us a distraction from why we are here. His mother crossly takes it away from him and ticks him off, which we find rather sad; but really and truly no one wishes to be here on Christmas Day. The stresses and strains are with us all. We take in to Rosie her twenty-four-year-old stocking which we have filled with a few small gifts and open it for her. She is completely unaware of anything, which day it is or what we are doing. I lean down towards her in an attempt to give her a hug and get caught in one of her lurching 'bedside to bedside' motions. As her left arm moves upwards, it unintentionally wraps itself around my neck and I hold her tightly to me for a few seconds before she pulls free and continues her familiar pattern of repetitive behaviour. Adrian snaps a photo of this as a reminder of today, a treasured moment, the first hug, albeit involuntary, that I have had since she came home just before her accident.

You lie here mute, morbid and misrepresented as I sit here crestfallen to my core. I have never felt such pain inside as I do now, my love, this happy time of year you love so much. If you could look up to my face as I peer over you and see my laughter lines, now altered to lines of pain, you would comfort me, I know you would – that bubbly, bouncy, beautiful YOU that I hunger and ache to have back in my life.

To pass the time during the morning, we hang a string of coloured light baubles over Rosie's bed. They seem to attract her empty, hollow gaze in fits and starts. As we occupy ourselves, we hear a booming "Ho ho ho!" as two or three members of the hospital staff dressed in Christmas outfits pop their cheery heads around the curtain to wish Rosie a 'Happy Christmas' and offer her a gift. As they eagerly wait for her to open it and anticipate some interaction, I find myself explaining to them through fumbled sentences that she is unaware of what's going on at the moment. This brings a hard lump to my throat and I choke back my tears. They retreat silently as I offer them a despondent "thank you".

ANTS IN MY BRAIN

We spend a few more hours with Rosie and leave her sleeping comfortably. Her favourite day of the year passes by without her. We too may choose to forget this particular Christmas.

On Boxing Day, we all breathe a bit of a sigh of relief that we made it through yesterday and that the day's over. With some tears and sadness, yes, but we made it; and we hope beyond hope that we will never have a Christmas Day like that again.

We go to see Rosie and spend some hours pampering her and making sure she is comfortable. At one point, she sits bolt upright as if startled by something, then slumps back down. It is good to see this movement again from her.

The day is wintry but dry and bright so the four of us decide to head out to Richmond Park for a brisk walk. It feels good to get a change of air and some exercise and it gives us a feel of the countryside. Up on the hill, we observe the park's majestic herd of deer sitting, almost in touching distance, as we amble along. The branches of the first humble catkin poke through, contrasting with the vast treescapes that blend amicably alongside their backdrops of concrete. It's a beautiful park and walking amongst many others with their dogs does us all the world of good and gives us a chance to temporarily empty our heads of hospital life. Will and Pollyanna talk about their studies and fill us in on general events that have helped to make their Christmas a little easier to bear.

Christmas to New Year week sees a marked change in staff numbers on the ward with not a great deal happening. It's a welcome break in some ways as everyone is appreciating these few 'low key' days and it means we can engage with the staff a little more in a light-hearted way.

Over the next few days my sisters pay a visit and see a real improvement in Rosie; and although she is still in a minimal conscious state, she is less poorly than she was when they last saw her in her early days on Intensive Care. She has few visitors apart from immediate family. Friends periodically ask to visit but she is in no fit state to see them and the shock could be too much for them. We hope we can give them the choice to see her in time.

Chapter 10

Facing the New Year with Hope

With Edd and Dani now returned from Sweden, they keenly encourage Adrian and me to visit them in Hertfordshire for a quiet and much-needed break over the New Year. After some persuasion we agree and head off in the comforting knowledge that our other offspring will pop in and visit Rosie on the day we are away. It's a welcome relief to be out in the countryside and to walk Monty again; and the change of air energises us. It gives us a chance to take stock a bit and enjoy, as much as we all can, some down time with Edd and Dani.

As we welcome in the New Year, the start of 2015, we feel a sense of positivity for the year ahead and plan to move forward with hope that we will see the change in Rosie's progress that we all crave. This is emphasised by the many good wishes from friends and family, bolstering our mood immensely.

We arrive back at the hospital on New Year's Day afternoon, refreshed mentally and physically from our break and ready to start our bedside vigil again. Rosie is still very restless and the staff keep her morphine at a level that keeps her comfortably out of pain. Are we imagining things, or is her awareness increasing? Her expression seems quizzical, as her eyes follow our movements a little more, giving us the impression that she recognises our faces but is unable to place us from her jumbled-up viewpoint. I keep my now well-trained roving eye on her intently, hungry to pounce on any change I might see.

It's five days after the New Year and finally the day has arrived for Rosie's teeth wires to be removed. It is wonderful to see her mouth open naturally again, even if rather tentatively as the sensation and pain seem uncomfortable. She will have to keep the metal bars on her upper and lower teeth for another week or two but even so, she looks more natural than she has done for weeks.

The staff are very happy to report to us that Rosie will now be able to transfer to Kent Ward tomorrow. This ward, on the third floor of the Atkinson Morley wing, is a neurological ward for acute patients and Rosie will stay here until, hopefully, she progresses through the Post Traumatic Amnesia (PTA) stage of recovery.

As we prepare for her move, I am encouraged by the staff to bring in some night clothes for her and I pop up to Tooting and pick her up some bright pink dog-patterned pyjamas and some multicoloured spotted nightdresses. She wouldn't normally have been seen dead in these, but I'm sure I am forgiven.

You would think it would be a normal and instinctive reaction to bring in night clothes for Rosie but because she has been in such a fragile state for so long, it's not easy to know where to start in the process of personalising her again, or how far to go. It's as if we have lost our ability to make these decisions as we have felt so out of control of anything up to this point. We are all learning on this journey of her rebirth.

Chapter 11

Move to Kent Ward

In preparation for her move to Kent Ward, Rosie's 'trachi' weaning begins now that her wires have been removed. It will be such a relief to see her rid of this large hose extending from her throat, and one less tube for her to attempt to pull out. Once the weaning transition has started, when tubes are removed and breathing returns to normal, a simple plaster is popped over the wound to protect it from infection until it heals and forms a scar. Rosie manages this brilliantly and within twenty-four hours we see her breathing normally again. This is a real step forward on the chart of progress. It's crazy to see her cough relatively normally now. No more avoiding the propelling mucus sprays when she has an infection, although we have a long, long way to go before we can observe her politely putting her hand over her mouth.

The transfer to the ward sees her placed in a small, bright single side room at the end of a long corridor with a large picture window overlooking the city. We fill the room with familiar ornaments from the bedroom in her flat: little pictures she may come to recognise in time and more photos of family and friends, as well as additional soft cushions for her bed to keep her comfy.

Rosie is not able to be on a more general ward with others just yet; her thrashing around, restlessness and totally unaware state would be difficult for other poorly patients to deal with. She is still pretty unwell and needs one-to-one care twenty-four hours a day in case she harms herself or falls out of bed.

As she settles into her new environment, we continue as we have been for the past two months with the daily routine of commands, familiar tunes and conversation, stimulating her as much as we can in short bursts in the hope of seeing a change or response of some kind.

Still nothing! Why nothing? What do we have to do to get you to communicate with us? My nightmares know exactly where that Putney hospital is. I have seen a room from its outside that I visualise you permanently in. A bed, soft sensory lights and lava lamps, like the one you used to have when they were all the rage. And the many long years have now passed, and I am still sitting, watching you as my older self, watching you but not you... that someone that I once knew...

It's Saturday, the end of the second week in January. All the family and their partners are here, bringing with them their usual and much-needed freshness and banter to the room. We prop Rosie up in bed and try to include her in our general upbeat conversation, hoping this may encourage a reaction from her of some sort. Normally Rosie would be very vocal at this point and full of chatter, and we reflect on the twenty-four years we have been trying to shut her up. Now we are so desperate to hear her voice again.

Dani has successfully engaged Rosie in looking at a family photo of her with her siblings and Monty the dog for longer than we have witnessed before. We feel she may be following what Dani is saying to her, if only briefly. Pet animals, we are told, have proved to be a huge aid in brain injury recovery. They often trigger emotions and speech amongst other things. We were told that a horse was recently brought into the grounds of St George's for its owner to see and the unique contact of human to animal really made a difference to the patient. We have asked if it is possible for Monty to be brought to the hospital so that Rosie can see him, in the hope of prompting her speech.

On a similar note: music, and the power it has over human emotion, never ceases to amaze me, particularly when we are in those dark and difficult times of our lives. From our large collection of 1970s and 1980s vinyl to our present-day online music streaming accounts, rearing our children on a diet of music went hand-in-hand with filling their bellies with good food. Rarely did a day pass without something blaring out of somewhere. It was a given, when the children needed to let off steam or be cheered up, that we would put some music on and dance around the rooms of the house like mad things. It was such a great antidote for everything. The teenage years were a competitive ground for sound, and mercifully they found the headphone sets!

For our family at the moment, any song played in a minor key plays havoc with our hearts and our tear ducts. One particular tune that's currently having a lot of radio play is Hozier's 'Take me to Church'. Hozier's haunting vocal sound accompanied by the powerful surges of his musical score hit us all right to the core, but the sombre lyrics are perhaps ones we choose not to investigate in too much detail. We hear it daily and this has since become our own powerful reminder of this time for us all. It brings us back instantly to this tiny room in St George's Hospital, never failing to fill to the brim our emotional quota, a signature tune to this very painful period of time.

Our daily lives have to function as best they can around the hospital visits. I choose to stay with Rosie all day, returning to her flat in the evening. Adrian now spends most of his week at work in Dorset, dropping Pollyanna off at her university in Winchester on his way home on Sunday and picking her up on Thursday. The other family members come to visit every weekend. We are establishing a pattern so that we can continue to keep all our lives outside the hospital on as even a keel as is possible.

This Sunday afternoon Will and I stay with Rosie when everyone leaves and, with only the two of us here, she suddenly seems to focus her attention on Will quite intently, gazing at him as if questioning who he is. Rosie has always been quite close to her younger brother in between the scraps and he has been very affected, as we all have, by what's happened to her. Will and I both get a strong sense that she knows who he is. She is particularly active this afternoon and is becoming quite vicious to us when we touch her, lashing out to pinch and scratch. Will may be allowed to think differently about her, after experiencing this, but we all understand it's par for the Post Traumatic Amnesia course, and as she is completely unaware of what she is doing we don't take it personally.

To help with this dilemma, the nurses have now strapped large boxing type gloves on her hands to help prevent her pulling at her food and pee tubes, and to protect us all from her scratches. She is starting to find her fighting spirit, we think!

I spend my days at the hospital and evenings back at the flat. I busy myself washing and drying Rosie's daily bag of pyjamas and other bits, lugging them to and from the laundrette that is, thankfully, just around the corner from the flat. I attempt to catch up on messages and phone calls but usually I am too exhausted to do anything that requires much effort. Lauren and I regularly chat over the day's events and keep each other company. It's not how it should be for either of us, but we make the best of things as they are for the time being.

For the time being... 'A Tale for the Time Being'. I have read that book; it has two narratives that run parallel with each other, two generations telling their stories. This is us, isn't it, 'for the time being'. My story I am living and yours, I observe every day, even though you don't know this. I long for you to tell me yours, how it is, what you see and feel from your minimal-conscious and disarrayed existence. Will you ever remember anything about this time?

It's very hard for both Adrian and me to be so regularly apart and for so long; we normally spend much of our days together, having passed only a handful of nights away from each other during our married life. This new life, this temporary existence, is so difficult but we treasure the times we have together and maintain this unexpected routine as best we can, supporting each other from a distance. This tests our marriage to the max and, in our case, has thankfully brought us closer together.

Today the rain spits hard as I walk over to the hospital. I grab my usual coffee and shortbread treat from the café outlet that's based in the main hospital reception, and the newspaper for the crossword to occupy me when I need a bit of distraction during my bedside vigil, and head up to the Kent Ward.

I have started a routine of walking to the hospital each morning from Southfields, weather permitting. This gives me some head space and daily exercise which helps me cope with the long and emotionally exhausting days at the hospital.

My route takes me through Wardle Park and onto the busy Garret Lane. I then continue through Earlsfield past shops and cafés, with people dashing this way and that in purposeful motion, chancing it across the road – lucky escapes for some, and for some not so lucky.

I regularly see tall, slim, blonde female runners pounding the pavements just as Rosie had done on countless occasions before her accident. These images stir my emotions, leaving me with such a sense of sadness as I think of her now and how her life and freedom changed in that fateful moment, that split second of time last November.

Will you ever run again, my love? Will you ever even walk again? I can't place the 'current you' here, along these roads, running like these others around me do. It came so naturally to you, so effortlessly. Your gazelle-like stance and your beautiful tall physique, that long blonde ponytail of yours swishing behind you in perfect rhythm with your pace. How were you not seen? What happened on that morning? Will we ever know the answer ...?

My mind frequently wanders as I walk along these pavements; it flits and daydreams as I go. I am reminded, on this occasion, of a time when I was at a rural Moroccan market where I observed a huge pile of mixed-up, worn-out shoes; and I remember thinking then of the stories they could tell and of the journeys they had taken, if only they could speak. It's odd how that memory has come into my mind; and my shoes, now quite well-worn from pounding the corridors and wards of St George's and the London streets, would surely have a tale to tell. I am in effect telling their tale right now.

I continue onto Blackshaw Road and, before entering the hospital grounds to my right, I pass the Lambeth Cemetery. I regularly see families here attending graves, giving them a routine tidy-up and replacing limp, dying flowers with fresh blooms. On occasion I see hearses with newly-bereaved families alongside freshly-dug graves ready to bury a loved one. I'm constantly reminded when I observe these sorry sights that however hard life is at this moment, I have my daughter alive; and whatever lies ahead, she has survived. For that, I will be forever thankful.

I sit beside Rosie's bed each day and this relieves the member of staff to attend to others' needs. I have daily interactions with her Multi-Disciplinary Team (MDT). Her Occupational Therapist and Psychologist put up a board with some simple orientation sentences which tell Rosie – if she is aware, that is – where she is, what day, month and year it is; and I repeat them to her regularly, willing her to respond. Her Speech and Language Therapist brings in a small pot of chocolate mousse and we watch as she tempts Rosie to open her mouth. She takes a little from the spoon, swallows it and licks her lips and teeth afterwards. This is so encouraging to see; and it helps the beginning process of improving her swallow reflex. These throat muscles haven't been used for nearly two and a half months and now need to be gently stimulated in order for Rosie to be able to eat and drink again. This is something we had no idea needed to be done. How much we normally take for granted when we are fit and healthy.

Rosie's physios regularly change her leg splints which are now much lighter and more manageable since her feet are now pretty near at right angles to her legs – their painstaking hard work that has been religiously undertaken since she was on intensive care has paid off. They now entrust me with changing her splints in their absence. I find this a challenge, as she is still moving and kicking quite haphazardly but, if I judge it right, I can manage to do it without too much difficulty.

Her neurology consultant is the voice of steadfast reason. She constantly presents us all with a calm and experienced 'air of hope and encouragement', assuring us that all we witness with Rosie is very normal for a patient in this transitional period. She is unable to give us any definite answers to any of our desperate and quite random questions. She tells us succinctly, "Rosie leads, and we all follow." Why should Rosie change the habit of a lifetime? We have always been running to catch up with her, as she lived life generally at ninety miles an hour! We just wish it was a bit faster than the zero miles per hour it feels like right now. Maybe her natural Taurean stubbornness has the upper hand and she will come back to us when she is good and ready.

Adrian is back and pleased to observe the current progress. Rosie is sitting, propped up for very short periods a little more often, and he is able to feed her some mousse which she takes; and we see her swallow improving. I even manage to give her mouth a gentle clean afterwards without being pinched or scratched, which is a bonus. This brings back to us those early memories of feeding solids to our four children during their babyhood. It seems crazy that many of the milestones we have been through four times before, we are now witnessing all over again with one of our children as an adult.

The max fax team come to check her teeth bars and agree they can be removed under anaesthetic the following week, which is great news. This will signify the end of their work and Rosie can be discharged from their duties now, apart from the odd follow-up appointment.

When we arrive today we find Rosie hasn't been given any liquid food. This is because she successfully managed to pull a glove from one of her hands and has attempted to dislodge her feeding tube from her stomach by gingerly teasing it through her nostril. Thankfully, the staff caught her in the act but, as a precaution, she has had to have an x-ray to establish exactly how far it may have moved. They report that fortunately it's still safely *in situ* and they have now given her a set of gloves which she can't remove; but this doesn't stop her trying.

We do like to remove these gloves from time to time when we are watching her and this seems to relieve her frustration and calm her to a degree. We decide to pop Rosie's glasses on to see if they help her focus a bit more as she is looking around and holding her gaze with more accuracy now, and for longer. To our utter amazement she very slowly and precisely takes them off with her right hand and carefully puts them back on again.

The physios are now starting to encourage Rosie to move more. She moves, with frustration, within the limited confines of her bed so they are interested to see what she would do if given the freedom of a larger area, so they take her to the gym which is based near the ward. There she will have a detailed assessment of her current physical and cognitive state so that goals can be set to aid her recovery.

We are unable to observe her during this as it could be too painful to hear what is being discussed; so the staff relay to us the general gist of what happened during the session. They laid her on a large, soft-cushioned area flat on her stomach and she managed to turn herself onto her back, her left side seeming more mobile than her more damaged right. A soft cushion was placed in front of her and she attempted to pull herself up onto it.

She hasn't the power in her brain and body to hold herself in any position for long or progress on her own to a kneeling or standing position. However, for us, it's good to hear about this. It's a good starting point to begin to help her increase her mobility and she may now be given regular sessions to help improve.

O... is for optimism
January 2015 – March 2015

Chapter 12
Mobile Phone Magic

At the weekend, when the family are with her, we constantly put our heads together to think of new activities to encourage Rosie to progress; and today, we decide to place her mobile phone into her hand to see what she will do. Her smart phone has always been her third hand, like it is for most people of her age; so we hope that this familiar electronic device will promote some recognition and connection deep within her brain.

To our utter amazement, she very slowly and carefully, with purpose, moves her spindly left index finger across the top of the phone to turn it off and on again. She then, using her right thumb with natural ease, slides the phone to the right to open and proceeds to open an app. This has us utterly spellbound as not only can she open the app, but she also knows exactly how much pressure to apply to the screen to do this. We eagerly tell her team this news and they are fascinated as they have never before seen anyone who cannot communicate or respond to simple commands do this. We all hold so much hope that this could be the start of her awareness increasing, if only she would start to talk.

Over the next day or two, we see more progress with Rosie and her phone. Edd makes a call to her and she slides the phone open and presses the green button to answer, then immediately presses the red button to end the call. She then opens her contact list and puts the phone to her ear as if to make a call.

The excitement we all feel at watching this progress is immense, almost spellbinding. Surely this must indicate that her brain has retained its hard wiring for these processes; and it gives us hope that more of her retrograde memory, the memory she had prior to her brain being injured, may still be intact. These bouts of brain stimulation seem to have promoted some physical activity, too, and she starts to move around the bed, the whole 360 degrees, sits up and attempts to put her legs through a gap in the bedsides as if to escape. It has been incredible for us all to witness and we sit, impatient and insatiable for more breakthroughs to occur. After these wakeful periods and, when her brain gets over-stimulated even for short bursts, Rosie fatigues very quickly and shuts down into sporadic episodes of sleep. Her brain needs to repair and to absorb little bits of information at a time, as this will aid the rewiring to take place around her damaged areas.

It's Sunday and Adrian's day to go home to Dorset. I dig deep to find strength for the week ahead, but I am encouraged by Rosie being more awake and responsive. This gives us all the impetus to carry on.

Before Adrian and Pollyanna set off, we play some familiar music to Rosie and observe her listening for short bursts. Her phone is placed in her hand again and we sit eagerly anticipating more action. Edd has sent her a Snapchat and Pollyanna indicates to Rosie to open it. She knows exactly what to press and holds the 'snap' down until it finishes its countdown – incredible!

We keep watch as Rosie moves towards the opening gap at the end of her bed again and she looks towards the ensuite toilet. Maybe she is connecting her bodily function with the need to use the loo, which she must have observed us using from time to time. She tentatively puts her scrawny feet on to the floor, and using the bed bars, attempts to heave herself up to a standing position. We are on hand to support her as she flops back down onto the bed. This is overly ambitious for her at this stage as she is far too weak to stand with no leg muscle or strength to hold herself up, her body too frail and her brain unable. We are not permitted to take her out of bed to use the loo as this manoeuvre is still too risky and, combined with our inexperience, could prove disastrous. She is far too frail and unable to stand, and her mended leg is still in the non-weightbearing period. She will have to continue with her catheter and bed changes until she can progress further, but staff are stretched, and she would need many to assist her. What's the old proverb? 'It's no good trying to run before you can walk.'

Somewhere, though, somewhere deep within her, there must be a determination and a desire to do these things. As she settles again, we question whether we can hear some vague and intermittent whispers from her lips but then doubt this, telling ourselves to stop letting our imaginations run too far ahead.

The week commences with Rosie having a general anaesthetic to remove her teeth bars. This makes her mouth look so much better and her teeth are able to be cleaned properly for the first time in over a month. They look just as they did before her accident. I still do as much of her personal care as I am able, cutting and filing her nails, massaging her hands and feet. It's hard to brush her hair as she gets very agitated.

Rosie sleeps through most of the days between periods of activity when there is only me for company, and while she does I ponder as to what might stimulate her to talk. I am currently reading an inspirational book written by an American brain scientist, who writes about her own journey through her stroke, observing her own mind through her understanding of the brain as it deteriorates and subsequently recovers after its injury. She documents her journey through her brain injury recovery; and her mother was instrumental in supporting her throughout. At one point, her mother lies beside her bedridden daughter and talks slowly to her, wrapping her arms around her and offering comfort and support as only a mother can.

I seriously consider this as I sit beside Rosie, for the closeness it may bring for us both and the stimulation it may encourage for her speech, but then selfishly cry off, choosing self-preservation since I might come off far worse from her punches and end up as an inpatient of St George's myself.

These days, these long days as I sit beside your bedside, the longing I have for you to recognise me is unbearable, the need for you to communicate so desperate. As I hang over your bedside, I gently cup your face with my hands and look into your eyes, willing your vacant expression to change and your eyes to fill with the warmth they once had. I sense you know I am with you and who I am. I cry to you as I talk softly and gently, the pain heavy with each tear that falls. I know you are 'locked in', I am convinced of that and I just don't have the key to get you out.

I have the idea of putting Radio One on to see if this might encourage Rosie to talk. Hearing Fearne Cotton's familiar voice seems to catch her attention and she listens intently. It's as if she needs to understand the process of how to talk again. I repeat this daily and I now deeply sense that she has latched on to something; her brain must be working hard to kick-start her speech again.

Each day, a little more progress is made towards Rosie's eating and drinking. She is now eating a whole pot of yogurt a day and we hope to expand this to other food and drink over the coming days and weeks. This proves to be the case as she progresses by swallowing tiny mouthfuls of puréed hospital food. This doesn't always go smoothly, and she spits it out in disgust a lot of the time. It's quite tasteless and bland, just like jars of processed baby food. It does make me chuckle to see the roast dinner: rounds of a puréed brown meat substance that are made to resemble slices, blobs of orange purée fashioned into the shapes of baby carrots. Perhaps this tempts the more aware patients but I can't think how. I do completely understand that this is purely a mechanical process to enable a patient's progression to eat again. The taste buds definitely have to take a back seat in this transitional period until proper food can be introduced.

As her throat is improving, we can now offer Rosie a plastic-covered beaker with a straw containing thickened squash to see what she does. She takes the cup from my hand with her left hand and clasps the straw with her spindly right fingers, moving it directly to her mouth and sucking up the liquid. This is so natural and almost effortless. We will have to offer Rosie continuous support with this for her to progress over the coming weeks so that she can eat enough food and drink to put on and retain weight – then, her feeding tube can finally be removed. Judging by the tiny amounts she is eating, this will take some doing. She is still quite emaciated and can't seem to gain any weight, as she has always had a fast metabolism. Perseverance will be the key.

Chapter 13

Where's Mum?

We are now into the last week of January 2015. Adrian and Pollyanna return for the weekend. We sit by Rosie's bed and encourage her to look in her handbag. She removes each item individually, examining the contents of her purse and opening her lipstick, and then carefully places everything back inside. She briefly flicks through a magazine, although with no evidence of reading anything or paying attention to the articles. As we sit beside her, she makes a husky cough and, after this, Pollyanna is convinced she hears the word 'cough' coming from Rosie's lips in a very low whisper. We now feel certain we are on the brink of change.

The following day we arrive at the hospital, intending to wash Rosie's hair and busy ourselves with the familiar care routines we have followed for the past months. As we enter her room, we see two or three nurses and carers surrounding her bed, already washing her hair.

Feeling a bit miffed at this scene, we reluctantly turn to go out and to wait until they have finished, only to be hastily beckoned back in. "She is starting to talk!" a nurse says eagerly. "Rosie pointed to the radio and said 'on' and to her head and said 'itchy', so that's why we are washing her hair!"

Tears of utter relief are shed by the three of us and some by the staff who regularly care for her. We stand aghast, hugging each other with sheer joy, not quite believing what we are hearing. It's like leaving your child at playschool only able to crawl and to come back having missed their first steps. As we stand in the doorway, a carer's raised voice penetrates through our sobs: "She also asked, 'Where's Mum?'" This sends me into a meltdown like never before. I sob and sob, months of pent-up anguish and pain pouring out in a matter of seconds. I shall never feel anything quite like this emotional release and joy for any moment ever again in my life; it was something so incredible, so precious, so valuable.

This is the stuff that only my dreams are made of, my love: this day, the day you said my name again and recognised me as your mother. Have you sensed that I have been by your side these past months, waiting for you? Have you? There is nothing more to add here now, for now you have said all that needs to be said ...

As whispers spread around the wing that Rosie is talking, we have visits from many of the staff who have had a connection with her in some form or another during her journey so far at St George's, ranging from many lovely carers to a paramedic who helped her on the day of her accident. From a janitor who developed a soft spot for her, even after regularly emptying her endless pee bags during the early days in intensive care, to the many nurses and care specialists who have all looked after her during the seventy-four days she has been an inpatient at St George's. They are as ecstatic as we are at this wonderful breakthrough; and the comfort and support they give us is overwhelming.

Throughout the rest of today, we sit hanging onto every one of her whispering words. She asks in simple language what's happened to her and where we are staying. We all have a celebratory cup of tea together, Rosie's thickened and drunk through a straw, with her announcing, "First cup of tea in a while," which made us laugh so much. We call the other family members during the day and continually keep them updated with every word she says.

Pollyanna asks her if she still likes her favourite sitcom *Friends* and she replies, "Of course I do;" and Adrian asks her if she wants to watch an Arsenal match, to which she replies, "I will watch it tomorrow."

We feed her a bit of her puréed curry supper and she says "spicy," indicating perhaps that she still doesn't particularly like spicy food. Lauren has now arrived and Rosie, looking at her, gently touches her arm and says, "Hello, how are you? I can't believe you have come here too!" This makes us all laugh. Lauren replies, "Actually, Rosie, I have been here with you quite a lot of the time; and how the hell are you!"

That evening we all go back to the flat armed with a bottle of champagne and together we celebrate, toasting with renewed confidence the beginning of Rosie's future. Our family and friends are doing much the same from wherever they are, as the many texts and photos fly back and forth. What a day it's been today.

We settle into bed emotionally drained but comforted that our hope is now renewed and the two possible paths of recovery that have been hanging over us like the grim reaper with his scythe have now become one. With the next phase tantalisingly within our sights, we are steering our course towards the Wolfson!

The weekend falls the day after this exciting development and we plan to go to Edd and Dani's overnight to celebrate, a family get-together which incorporates Edd's birthday celebrations too. We visit the hospital before we head off and find Rosie exhausted and irritable after such a big day yesterday. Now she is starting to vocalise, she adds swearing to the mix of hitting and pinching, all still part of the Post Traumatic Amnesia stage she is now well and truly entering. She tells Adrian to "f*** off", digging her nails into his arm and hitting him as hard as her weakness allows. We don't worry, as it's just wonderful to hear her say anything; and our bruises will heal.

We return the following afternoon, refreshed and still very much fuelled with elation, and the staff tell us that Rosie has had her first full night's sleep since the 10th of November last year. She is chatting – garbled, mostly whispered sentences – so we try to decipher the more lucid comments. She gesticulates to me that she wants my cup of tea and KitKat so I offer her a little tea and a smidgen of chocolate, still aware that she might choke, as she has yet to try solid food of any sort. We ask her to point to a photograph of Monty and she does.

We set about issuing Rosie with the same commands we have been using for months while waiting for a response, and now she is reacting to them all – we are ecstatic. We duly omit the 'pen pushed down on her cuticles' and the 'hefty pinching into her clavicle' that would just be too mean. My guess is we leave that bit for her to do to us now with her pinching and biting gestures – perhaps she is getting her own back.

Just before her supper, she pulls my arm towards her and whispers in my ear, "What's for firsts?" "Well, I would rather not tell you, Rosie, but just enjoy those carrot shapes." Nom nom. We hope that over the next few days she can make the transition from puréed to semi-solid food.

Rosie gave us her first smile today, which knocked us all for six; and we all behave like children in a sweet shop, waiting in anticipation for the next 'sugar hit' of progression to happen.

Your smile, your beautiful, sunny smile. You could always light up a room with that one, your key asset to cheer up a dreary day or make a sad someone happy again. How delighted you have made us all seeing this again, my love; a smile says so much and, slowly, steadily, you seem to be coming back to us from an empty place that none of us will ever know, not even you.

At the moment, all Rosie's sporadic speech is in whispering sounds so her speech and language therapist encourages her to develop deeper sounds to help stimulate her vocal cords into action, as she fears they may have been damaged a bit over the course of her time here. The months of lack of use have all added to their deterioration. Rosie's current voice is nothing like it used to be.

This is something we find very amusing, as Rosie has always had the loudest of shouts and cannot shout at all now. Her sentences are quite muddled but she instigates chats and throws into the now standard 'topsy-turvy' conversation words like 'Glastonbury' and 'ferry trips', indicating that she may remember festival experiences and family holidays somewhere deep in her memory.

We had some great family holidays in France; always a little unconventional, I suppose. Our ancient, gas-converted Land Rover Defender was always full to the brim with children, camping gear, bikes and the signature nappy bucket. A standard black silage sheet was always on hand to cover and protect the bulging roof rack, should it rain. We would always find a campsite with enough space for our large but simple tent and actively explore the French way of life for the week we were away. We survived then on a small agricultural wage, so holidaying was always on a shoestring budget. One of the main highlights was our excursions to the hypermarkets; the French do these so well. Finding interesting food to cook up on our little two-ring camping stove was great fun, and we were always amazing ourselves by how we could feed our growing family so simply. We cycled the beautiful countryside, swam in pools and rivers and drank lots of delicious, cheap wine. They were good times.

I look back with such fondness on these memories, as I know you always did. I say 'DID' as I don't know yet if you will be able to remember any in detail, if at all. Life was quite simple then. I am glad not to have been able to see far into the future and to your adult years. I am not sure I could have prepared myself for this, let alone have prepared you.

Rosie has always been a very sociable person, and in between the swearing and pinching episodes, she politely says hello to the staff when they come to care for her. She frequently asks them how they are, which is hilarious.

Her constant sporadic movements seem to have calmed down now and are a little more fluid, which is good to see. She now has periods of time in the day without her boxing gloves, although she is still permanently observed night and day as her behaviour continues to be quite erratic. I still give her phone to her daily and, on taking a closer look, I see that she has interestingly opened her Map-My-Run app, the app she always used to monitor her running performance, which we find intriguing. Has she clicked on that last fateful run and, if she has, what is she thinking, I wonder?

Now Rosie is a little more aware of night and day, she asks us many times when we are about to leave, if she can leave the hospital and come home with us. She tells us repeatedly, "I'm fine" and "I'm normal;" and when we ask her what she has been doing, more often than not she replies, "I've been upstairs." The next floor up is the helipad on top of St George's – not sure if that's really the best place for you, lovely, particularly as it's winter; you would freeze, dressed only in your Primarni-best PJs.

Chapter 14
Low after the High

Over the next few days we see a slight downward turn in Rosie's progress and this we are told can sometimes happen after a sudden upward surge of change. She catches a nasty stomach bug and is quite poorly from this, tending to sleep a lot more, and she is much less interactive with us. She behaves in a very childlike manner, pointing at everything and refusing to speak. Her consultant has concerns that she may have developed a stomach ulcer from the weeks and weeks of tube feeding so suggests she have an x-ray to check this and, as she is eating very little, there is talk of inserting a stomach peg via her lower abdomen to feed her.

This has left us feeling very flat as we know the Wolfson rehabilitation unit won't accept her if she is not eating normally; and once inserted, the stomach peg has to remain in for at least six weeks. Her consultant also requests a brain scan to see if there is any deterioration due to this slump in her progress after the initial upward and positive turn.

Thankfully, news from these procedures is positive, no further damage occurring in her brain and her stomach is fine. We are reassured that this is all part of her entering this new stage of her metamorphosis, and this is indicated in her behaviour sometimes as she calls the nurses 'the mums'. I am reminded that at her old school the lunchtime assistants were often referred to as 'the mums' or 'the grans' so perhaps her childhood will be the starting point of her new emerging self. I guess we have some idea of how to build on this as parents as she recovers but, as she is now very much an adult, it will be in a very different way to how it was the first time around.

My washing increases daily as Rosie develops a painful urine infection; she continually tries ways to get out of her bed, always indicating towards the loo as she becomes more aware of her needs. I just wish I was able to start helping her there; it would feel so much more dignified for her.

The decision is made to remove her catheter and encourage a bed pan, thus easing the obvious pain from her infection; and this is a small start to her regaining her capability in this function.

Each evening I leave St George's with Rosie's hospital bag containing 'pee-flavoured washing' and head up through the dark and bustling streets of Tooting to catch my usual bus back to Southside followed by a walk back to the flat. On my daily travels, I often witness a lot of kindness in our wonderfully cosmopolitan capital: little gestures from one to another which can sometimes go unnoticed with the hard and fast pace of life here. Maybe it's due to my emotional antenna being on full alert that I feel more sensitive than normal to others around me. I spent time living and working in London in the early '80s and chose to move back to the West Country. I could never have imagined I would be back again years and years later in circumstances such as these, circumstances that have started to become such a familiar part of my life.

The buses are always crowded at this time of night so I often wait in line for one on which I may have a chance of a seat, making the choice not to stand 'cheek by jowl' with other commuters and squashing my washing bag too close for fear of them thinking it's me who has wet myself. As I sit silently with my own life story, observing the many human beings around me, I ponder on the lives that exist behind each exterior I see: a variety of narratives, perhaps many far worse than my own. I sometimes observe other women, mothers maybe, glancing down on occasions at the standard patient hospital bag I carry, then looking at me as if wondering too. I long to ask for a hug from one of them, for some solace of some kind, a kindred spirit to talk to through all the turmoil and angst I feel at this moment in time.

You should be on these buses, my love, not me. Returning from your day's work to your little flat in Southfields, not me. This London life is yours, not mine. It's not of my choosing but I am coping the best I can. I think you would be proud of me; I hope so. Coping is all I have come to know amid these circumstances. We are good at coping, us mothers; it's what we do best, I guess.

Over the next few days Rosie starts to perk up a bit and interactions start again. We are informed by the staff that she asks for Adrian and me when we are not there and seems much happier, waving and smiling to those around her. Her general demeanour is still very stilted, and her eyes can appear very glazed, particularly when she is fatigued. She is a shadow of her former self but we see the tiny sparks of her personality appear from time to time which we cling to in the hope that she regains as much of herself as possible over time. The physios are regularly getting her into her chair now and taking her out of her bedroom setting for a little spin, which is good. We keep our fingers crossed that the orthopaedic team will give the go-ahead for her to weight-bear on her right leg soon, now that the repairing and healing have taken place.

We accompany the physios as they wheel Rosie down to the ground floor of the hospital for her first jaunt away from the ward. We sit outside the Peabody's café for a short period and she glances around continuously, taking in this bustling environment for the first time. Her gaze flits from moment to moment, unable to concentrate for more than a second on any one thing; and her very mixed-up sentences are whispered, which makes her hard to understand; but she is cooperative and calm.

Back in her room, we start to try and orientate Rosie, testing her memory by asking her the month and date. She replies, "April 5th" when in reality it's the end of January. This leaves us wondering what progress she will have made by this date in a couple of months' time. I hug her goodnight and she pinches my nose, still indicating that to get too close may not be such a good thing just at the moment.

Edd and Dani come this weekend and encourage Rosie to write something. She loosely grips the pen and writes her name in a very scruffy manner, similar to that of a child learning. She slowly reads out the title of a magazine and this gives us hope that her reading and writing skills, however sketchy, are still intact. The start of relearning these fundamental skills is now a possibility. Rosie asks me for her Vaseline, which she carefully smears onto her lips. She would once never go anywhere without this so this little routine has clearly stayed with her. She is now drinking from a mug; the contents are still thickened, but the progress away from a child's beaker and a straw is encouraging.

During a lengthy meeting, Rosie's psychologist mentions some interesting facts. Just to complete the process of picking up an apple and taking a bite out of it involves the human brain in thousands of tiny processes, ranging from firstly knowing what to do with the apple, to the hand-eye coordination of bringing it to the mouth; then exerting the correct pressure to hold the apple; plus the complex chewing and swallowing processes. Each and every bit of progress in the right direction, however small, is so positive for the future.

I decide to go back home to Dorset with Adrian today, Sunday, for the first time since my overnight visit in early December; it's now early February. I am quite exhausted and in desperate need to recharge.

As we drive through Dorset across the undulating Askerswell hills towards Bridport, I glance over through the farmland gaps towards the glinting sea, the sun tenderly touching its surf at selected points. I so desperately want to believe our own tide has turned for us now, to be reassured that we can start to put trust in the hope we have had for so long.

Being home feels very strange to me and it's as if I only exist somewhere else now. The house is suffused with a musty, unlived-in odour; and Monty's absence underlines the strangeness. Adrian just carries out the basics, existing through those workdays during the week. I can't bear to think of him sitting alone each evening and enduring the long journeys to and from the capital, just as he can't bear thinking of me coping alone in London. But it's what we both have to do to cope and to get by, each doing our bit to hold the tentative threads of our life together. I feel so aimless here and, as I move from room to room, I arrive at the kitchen. I open our normally full fridge and scan its now sparse contents, trying to drum up some enthusiasm to cook. I casually spot some very mouldy dips that had been left by Pollyanna and Will when they came home for a brief visit to see friends before Christmas. This tiny, pathetic incident sets me off; I sit down at the kitchen table and weep in desperation.

The next day I take a solitary walk around the frosty grounds of the caravan park, and its emptiness shouts back at me, echoing exactly the way I feel. I try desperately to reconnect in some way with the life I left behind here in November last year.

Under these circumstances, we need to find some way of making my own life function as best it can, so Adrian and I hatch a plan. It might be good for me to come home with him each Sunday afternoon and catch the train from Axminster back up to London on the Tuesday morning, allowing me enough time to visit Rosie for a few hours each Tuesday afternoon. This way I will only be missing one day away from her but equally, for my own personal wellbeing, having some home time will recharge my batteries enough to enable me to carry on. We need to initiate a pattern for ourselves, to take regular short breaks from the long and draining weeks spent at the hospital. Our conversation is inevitably always centred around Rosie and the hospital; so a regular night away at home should offer a little distraction.

I agree, although reluctantly at first, as I struggle with the prospect of leaving Rosie; but I know in my heart that I must do this, to somehow bridge this old life with the new. I call the hospital to see how Rosie is, to be told that, in her agitation, she has pulled her glove off and managed to extract her feeding tube through her nose and out of her stomach; she has had to go to theatre and be sedated for this to be reinserted. I push away the guilt and try not to beat myself up for not being there to keep an eye on her.

I arrive at the hospital late on Tuesday afternoon from Dorset. Always desperate for a pee, I use the loos at the entrance of Atkinson Morley wing. These loos always have a pleasing scent of peaches. It's funny how little things like this can give you some comfort, and the familiarity jolts me into the present and I immediately slot back into hospital life.

It will take time to get used to this new routine and I feel a sudden sense of guilt on seeing Rosie after a day's break. I am relieved, though, to find her quite awake after her anaesthetic yesterday and quite chirpy too. She calls me 'Emma' which tickles me – where did that come from?

There has been an improvement in her vocal sound, and I can actually hear her faint voice now instead of the whispering sounds we usually strain to hear. Rosie repeats over and over again the phrases "Everything is normal," "Everything is fine." I am not quite sure if I could entirely agree with her on this point and try to encourage her into broader conversation.

After giving Rosie her phone to amuse her, I realise she has opened two apps: Google maps and BBC weather in Tooting. This makes me wonder if she is secretly plotting her escape. Some patients do try to do this whilst in this unpredictable PTA stage and I would not put it past her.

During the week, I decide to bring in some homemade 'spag bol' to encourage Rosie to eat a bit more. A little of her favourite homemade food might stimulate her taste buds and some memories, too. We sit in the patients' day room and consume our lunch together, despite her protests about her throat being sore. She is having to learn to eat again and maybe this semi-solid food makes her feel frightened and fearful of choking; and she is perhaps in some discomfort as the food passes down her very sensitive gullet.

The dinner ladies loved you at primary school, always eating up the left-over cabbage and custard. Once you ate fish pie for breakfast before school, even though porridge and eggs were on offer. We have always joked about this. Food has always been important to our family, hasn't it, never wasting anything and always thinking up ways to use up leftovers – if there were any leftovers, that is. You loved baking, didn't you, making cakes for your work friends on their birthdays. Can you draw these memories to mind now? Any of them? Have they been wiped out now, with the ease of an eraser swiping over a whiteboard full of words, leaving in its wake a blank and barren canvas?

Chapter 15

Our Butterfly Emerging

When I arrive today, Rosie is fresh from her first proper shower since her accident. The staff have washed and plaited her hair, which seems to have perked her up.

The plan today is to see if Rosie is able to take any steps. I witness her weight-bearing for the first time, even though she is totally unable to stand alone unsupported. The physios hold her in an upright position, supporting her on either side as she takes very small, tentative shuffles up the ward corridor. It takes a long while as she has to stop to refocus due to the constant distractions. She consciously needs to think about each step, putting one foot in front of the other, and the evident fatigue hinders her pace. We feel encouraged that she can still remember how to do this and it's evident her brain is working very hard to coordinate this process; and she rests for the remainder of the morning. This exercise has to be repeated time and time again for little improvements to be made but, thankfully, the long challenge of learning to walk again has finally begun.

Adrian and Pollyanna arrive at midday and we all sit with Rosie in the day room and have lunch together. Rosie repeats herself constantly, still unable to hold any new information for much more than a second or two, asking questions over and over again – for instance, when am I visiting, and at what time. The need for frequent reassurance, as her brain rewires, gets very wearing at times but we continue to reiterate exactly what she wants to hear and whenever she wants to hear it.

Rosie's neuro psychologist offers us a simple explanation as to how the brain rewires. When a brain injury occurs, it's similar to picking up a filing cabinet and emptying the contents onto the floor. Both events happen in an instant; both can take a long time to be carefully put back together again, or near to their original order. Damaged brains can have billions of severed neurons after an impact, but the brain has a unique way of creating different pathways around its damage to rewire itself; and this is called neuro plasticity. I have interpreted this reference as my 'ant analogy', as ants replicate this very well. We had times on family holidays when we would sit and observe an ant (the neuron) carry a small piece of baguette up a wall or over an obstacle, trying every which way to manoeuvre it, working down a path, finding a blockage and going back to start again a different way, often enlisting support from its helpers. It travels over and around obstacles (brain damage) to eventually reach its final destination. I like to think this is a simple way to understand this long and challenging process. Brains continually work down many different pathways to rewire, just as ants do in their desire to achieve their goal; and we have helpers, too.

Rosie's complete disorientation as to where she is continues to make us all laugh, not least herself. She reveals that last night she had apparently been staying at her Nan's house in Padstow – that must have been a flying visit.

As Rosie sits, engaged in befuddled conversation with Pollyanna, she pulls one of her typical sisterly faces at something Pollyanna says and gives her a mocking smile. It's wonderful to see these signs of her sense of humour emerging together with some distinctive elements of her personality, those well-rehearsed exchanges of sibling connection peeping through.

As we sit drinking our cups of hospital tea, Adrian starts to tap his fingers rhythmically on the table. Rosie observes him briefly before joining in. Before long they are both rapping loudly on the table, causing Rosie to laugh out loud, really enjoying the fun; and we all giggle together at yet another great moment, her sense of fun shining through as it always did.

We were told in the early days to expect someone completely new to emerge after a brain injury, someone with different personality traits and certainly not the person they once were. They might behave oddly, have strange food tastes and even, in some cases, a different accent. This has frequently been a worry at the back of our minds: the very thought of grieving for the person we love and welcoming a new person back into our lives seems far too much of an adjustment to contemplate. We believe the best thing we can do is to act as normally as possible towards Rosie, making her feel comfortable and relaxed in our familiar company. This is sometimes easier in theory than in practice, but by taking this approach we hope to bring out as much of the old Rosie as we can; and so far, this seems to be working.

Continuing with this idea and with the family visiting over the weekend, we decide to recreate a family Sunday lunch in the day room. We arrange a time that's agreeable to the staff, falling after the main hospital lunchtime period. I make a large cottage pie for us all which we are given permission to reheat in the ward kitchen. Sadly, no wine is permitted to accompany our meal, so we have to make do with hospital water on this occasion. This brings a rather abstract feeling of one of our Sunday lunches complete with the usual banter but in the most unusual of settings. It does give Rosie the chance to sense what it feels like to be part of a family mealtime again and prompts her to eat a little more, which was one of the positives we hoped for. She seems to enjoy the occasion and it feels good for us all to be together.

After lunch, we decide to give Rosie a trip out of the ward and meander down to the wing's foyer for a change of scenery. We wheel her to the entrance and outside for a short moment, her first taste of outside air since that early morning run last November. The change in temperature immediately affects her and she starts to shiver violently. We promptly go back inside, not wanting her to catch cold, but aiming to improve these short bursts of acclimatisation to the outside world over the coming weeks.

Edd takes charge today of Rosie and her chair, and with his love of wheels and his boisterous wickedness, he starts winding Rosie from side to side and at speed up the hospital corridors towards her ward. She absolutely loves this and tells him to stop (but don't stop) through her laughter. We all join in, sniggering at this hilarious scenario of Edd whizzing his brain-injured, heavily amnesic sister in her wheelchair at speed up and down the corridors of St George's. We hope no one is looking but feel sure that those who have come to know us and see no harm done would be secretly laughing from their offices and wards. We all leave at points during the afternoon, and Rosie, exhausted from her busy day, goes back to her bed for a well-earned rest.

You enjoyed today, I know you did, my love, I could see it in your eyes, your smile, your mien. We are all impatient now for you to come back to the YOU we know. In your still fragile state, I have no idea just how long this will take or what adjustments we will all have to make. So far you are doing great; all these little steps give us hope for you. I believe you feel this sense of belief seeping from us all, too.

I am always grateful to see my own bed for a couple of nights and although my sleep is often restless, and my time at home relatively unproductive, it gives me the chance to rest and recuperate from my exhaustion as much as I can. I call the hospital for an update just as Rosie happens to be passing by the reception desk in her chair and I chat to her briefly. The usual questions dominate the conversation but it's good to hear her upbeat voice as she is kept busy going to and from her therapy sessions and her mealtimes in the day room.

She is now having more regular therapy sessions. To add to her physiotherapy, she has psychology, speech and language therapy and her neuro occupational therapy team adjusts these in line with her progression. Her brain is incredibly muddled as she is still very much in a state of prolonged Post Traumatic Amnesia so it's very much a case of little and often, adapting to see what works and what doesn't.

I take my usual long Tuesday train journey back to the city. Sometimes my anxiety level can feel quite high on my travels and with it a sense of loneliness can kick in too. I have found a way to combat this by imagining I am carrying my children around with me on my shoulders and, with them, my beautiful grandma too. It helps to feel they are with me when I travel around on the trains and buses. It gives me encouragement to keep strong and to feel that I am not so alone.

I arrive at the hospital and the physios update me with the news that Rosie had spent five minutes exercising in a 'chair type' exercise bicycle. This is the first step towards getting her mobile again and her coordination and stamina are now being put to the test. They continue to encourage Rosie to practise her walking as much as she is able. Building the non-existent muscles in her legs will have a profound effect on her body's stability. She is still very fragile and wobbly and it takes so much of her energy to walk, even supported by two physios; but the more she does, the more she will improve. So we all start to help her walk up and down the longer hospital corridors, particularly at the weekend when the whole family are here. We start to record these walks on our phones so that in time she will be able to look back at the progress she has made. Rosie always seems to enjoy these challenges and chats nonstop, repeating the limited loop of questions she has stuck in her head over and over again. She giggles, laughing at her own chaotic condition as she goes.

Over the next week, the occupational therapist suggests we have a mini outing to the hospital café on the ground floor for afternoon tea and cake. I am asked to bring in some of Rosie's clothes for her to wear for the occasion and it's nice to see her in familiar day clothes again, even though they are swimming on her thin body.

As we wheel her up to an empty table, I observe her unease at being in this rather confined social situation for the first time. She still chats away, repeating the same sentences time and time again, with me repeating my answers. The longing I have for her to be able to retain more information in her memory gets progressively more frustrating. I crave the possibility of us both enjoying these sorts of experiences the way we used to; this longing is painful in my heart. But at the same time, this is a memory for me to treasure. I would have cut off my right arm in return for a moment like this only weeks ago; and look at us now.

Do you remember the little makeshift café you and Pollyanna made in the old barn on the farm? Plates of soggy mud and bits of wood served as food, garnished with crumpled leaves and blades of grass? I would sit, amid the trees, on the gnarly wooden stumps in the outside seating area you created and pretend to enjoy your cake and drink your tea. And the walks after school across the Yarty fields to beautiful Beckford Bridge with our tea picnics? We played Poohsticks and paddled in the icy water, swimming when the warmer summer months arrived. Your imagination had no bounds then; freedom was its fuel. Can you imagine anything now, bring to your mind these images to reminisce about?

Chapter 16
Friends Start Visiting

After discussions with Rosie's team we decide it's now time to reintroduce some of Rosie's old friends. Lauren has been visiting her from the start with the family. She has been unexpectedly thrust into our situation and has demonstrated her resilience and support in a way that few friends could have done, but she needs some respite herself now. Others have been keen to visit for some weeks; and now that Rosie is communicating, she will perhaps be more able to cope with this introduction of more visitors. Her two oldest school friends make the journey from Lyme Regis to see her and thankfully, she recognises them and interacts a little. It's not easy for anyone who has known her for so long to see such a shocking change in her, but they are encouraged, despite Rosie being quite aggressive at times. She tells us all to 'f*** off' and calls us all sorts of rude names. It must be seeing her school friends that's triggered this schooltime potty-mouth behaviour. As I suffer from occasional inappropriate laughter, it is sometimes hard not to laugh at this and I find myself continuously apologising to all the staff. They reassure me they have seen it all before, so nothing shocks them.

Now Rosie is holding herself more upright in her chair, we regularly sit for periods in the large and airy ward day room along with other patients for as long as her attention span permits. We still exchange the regular snippets of mixed-up conversation, whatever comes into her vague and muddled mind; and she chats continuously.

She is convinced she saw my sisters at home in Dorset last week and is certain, at least for this brief moment, that she is staying in a hotel. We go along at her slow and confused pace, subtly correcting her with the missing gaps of her lost time by mentioning why she is here and what she has been doing. Little or nothing is retained and most of her limited sentences are just repeated.

She now has short regular evening visits from her close friends, many of whom have worked with her in their Topshop days in Exeter and moved to London around the same time as she did to study and pursue their careers here. They know her very well and recognise many of her familiar personality traits re-emerging, her wicked sense of humour being one of these. Rosie makes them all laugh with her constant chatter and they all say she is like herself but on a very drunk night out; and there have been many of those over the years. These happy memories of her youth we hope will come back to her over time, perhaps with some of the more 'head down the loo' moments best left forgotten.

Rosie loves having them visit for company but at this stage can't remember who has been and when. We encourage her to write their visit times in a large 'week to view' diary and this proves the start of her using this as a simple memory aid. It helps to orientate her with the date and the days of the weeks and gives her something to keep focused on. We add our visiting times to her diary and the times of her regular therapy sessions, noting the names of the staff and the therapies they carry out. Rosie always insists on keeping it with her and constantly checks and rechecks the information in it, trying hard to retain even a tiny bit. She always had a very procedural way of working so it's a good indication that she may still work in this way.

Chapter 17

Bye-bye, Nasogastric

Now that Rosie has progressed to a semi-solid diet, she is eating more and gaining weight; and we are told that her nasogastric feeding tube can finally be removed, after thirteen long weeks. It's so wonderful to see her face free from this tube that had been so altering her looks. A great step. We can now erase the threat of the dreaded stomach peg completely from our minds and move forward.

With her awareness increasing, she has now progressed to being fully continent, although she needs help as she is still very weak and unable to stand on her own yet. I assist her regularly with this and most days we encounter some entertaining toilet moments where I have had to save her from falling into the loo, usually as a result of us both laughing too much.

These areas of progression have happened relatively quickly and it's hard to keep pace at times. It's quite staggering to think she is now medication-free as well, when we had imagined she would be on medication for life.

We all start to wonder if she will be able to move to the rehabilitation centre and our questions are answered during a family meeting. Adrian, Edd, Pollyanna, Will and I all attend this milestone family meeting, and Rosie's skilled therapy team update us as to her progress within their disciplines. Her consultant talks us through the next steps forward. Very soon Rosie will move into a six-bed bay on the same ward to get her used to socialising with other patients. We are all slightly apprehensive about the outcome of this as she is still very much in the Post Traumatic Amnesia stage so can display some random behaviour at times. Once the team are satisfied that she is well enough, she will be transferred to the Wolfson rehabilitation unit in St George's to continue her recovery. We are told by her psychologist that she is a bit of an anomaly since she performs well in some maths and language tests but is really poor on her short-term memory recall. Physically she is improving, and this can progress now if she continues to work hard.

We all make a visit to the Wolfson rehab unit. The pallid walls of this old centre are stark and the general decor unyielding; it has the markings of an archaic psychiatric hospital. We try to discount our uneasy observations and focus more on the opportunities there will be here for Rosie. We feel incredibly fortunate that Rosie can access this centre as part of our NHS. In America the private costs for rehabilitation can amount to thousands. The importance of good, consistent rehabilitation after brain injury can often be underestimated. Families bear the brunt of this as it can be difficult for people to access the often-sparse services offered within their areas. The Wolfson is one of the leading UK neuro rehab units, skilfully headed up by Rosie's consultant, and we are immensely privileged that she is able to access this facility.

Over the next few days, the transition from her small side room to a larger bay proves quite a challenge for

Rosie and she takes time to settle into this environment, becoming irritable at times and frustrated that she is in hospital (in the brief moments when she remembers where she is). Rosie continually asks Pollyanna to pack her bags for her so that she can go home, trying to get her on her side to dream up ways to escape. A primary school memory of Rosie, successfully persuading Pollyanna to 'bunk off' their after-school French club together, springs to my mind.

I found you both, eventually, meandering slowly up the leafy church lane which leads to the fields across from home. You both stop and stoop down together. I shocked you; you had no idea how worried I was then. You showed me the poorly bird with its broken wing that had drawn your attention. We decided to take it home and care for it in the warmth of our old Rayburn; the poor little thing didn't survive. You may not have had your French lesson, but we had a valuable and impromptu lesson of nurture within nature that day.

To make her transition to the bay a little more comfortable, I buy Rosie a duvet, some bright butterfly-printed covers and some new bits for her bed area. This immediately makes a difference to her little space and brightens the gloom of the hospital ward. We fill a new snack box with her favourite treats and magazines to keep her amused and connected with the celebrity gossip. These seem to initiate a reconnection with old memories of the stars she admires, bringing her a little more in touch with the outside world. Not needing to replace the magazines on a regular basis proves quite cost-effective, as at this stage she mostly forgets what she has read.

Getting her night and day routines reinstated is such a big part of normality but it takes time for this to happen within the hospital setting. The constant noise and milieu of the busy ward makes it almost impossible to sleep well. The staff gradually introduce morning and evening personal care routines and Rosie starts to take some responsibility for these herself, her carer keeping a watchful eye.

With the anticipation of warmer temperatures, progress has been made with getting Rosie acclimatised to the outside and I wheel her, pretty much daily, up to the café that's situated at the main entrance to the hospital. It's good to have regular tea and cake outings now and the more we do this the more she seems to feel at ease with the social setting, although it's difficult to command her attention for long due to the distracting busyness of the café.

Getting her used to the contrasts of outside and inside is still a challenge as going from the artificial warmth of the ward to the cold air of outside sends her body temperature regulator into a state of shock. We pile blankets and coats around her to protect her.

Rosie's godmother is visiting her today and, as we go out and about on our daily expedition, we happen to bump into some of the intensive care nurses who encourage us to take Rosie back to see everyone on the intensive care unit – they are so surprised with her progress and to see her so chatty and friendly. She has no idea where she is, no memory of her critical time spent here, and for that we are relieved. It's wonderful to see all the staff again and we make a pledge to do this when we can over her recovery period so that the staff can see her progress, the rewarding fruits of their challenging work and dedication. As one member of staff asks me for my email address, Rosie pipes up and articulately reels it off to them. We are amazed – why can she recall this instantly and still get confused as to where she is and why she is here? We still have a lot to learn about the memory in this complex brain system.

The emotional details of our time here are etched on the body of my subconscious mind. I will revisit that place at some point in the future. I can't begin to poke around in that space I so vehemently defend just now; the pain would knock me off kilter and I might crumble. I can't afford to crumble, not yet...

Chapter 18

Post Traumatic Amnesia Antics

With winter nearly at its end, the thought of springtime waiting in the wings, bringing with it much-needed colour to the dank winter earth, raises my spirits. I arrive today to find Rosie sitting on her bed in her familiar crossed-legged position, flicking through her magazines. She has always been a very flexible person and, as her limbs improve with activity, some of her natural poise starts to return. She now wears her ordinary clothes each day, recognising some that I have brought in for her from her flat and attempting to familiarise herself with the new ones I have purchased for her. She has straightened her hair and put on a little makeup with the help of her carers. It's so encouraging to see her looking more like herself, chatting and interacting with other patients.

We are always on the lookout for any marked behaviour changes resulting from her brain injury and always feared that with Rosie's sociable and extrovert disposition, her premorbid awareness and internal filter system could be exacerbated to include overly friendly and possibly anti-social behaviour.

One particular man on the ward is very loud and overfamiliar, continually walking around and displaying quite challenging behaviour. Rosie acknowledges his actions as not quite right and she mentions to us that he is invading her personal space when he comes close. We are relieved to hear her say this, indicating that she is making the choice not to get caught up in his antics and reaffirming to us that her social awareness and intuition are still present to some degree.

Each day sees little increments of progression despite Rosie forgetting moment to moment what's going on. Her personality continues to sneak through and we still have our increasingly entertaining conversations on a daily basis about where she thinks she is and what she has been doing. Today she thinks she has been at home swimming in the caravan park swimming pool. She asks where her car is and is convinced she has driven it recently.

She achieves a mile cycle on the chair bike and soon progresses to a proper exercise bike. After six minutes of cycling it's very clear to see how being upright and attempting more challenging exercises affects her brain and her stamina in a big way and she must rest and repair after each session.

At her physio sessions, Rosie manages a few steps on her own with the aid of rails for the first time and, when the family are here, we continually take her for little supported walks inside the hospital which we record on our phone cameras. These serve as significant reminders for us, particularly when we think progress is slow, as to how far she has come, and they will be good for her to look back upon. Rosie now wears trainers to do this which makes a difference; she walks more consistently and wobbles less. These old trainers resemble large blobs of ice cream at the bottom of those skinny stick-thin legs which look ready to snap at any given moment.

Rosie laughs at herself and continues to push through her walking with such determination, entertaining us and herself with her constant chatter in the process. As the warmer weather approaches it has become much easier to take her outside in her chair and we hope soon to be able to encourage her first steps outside the hospital doors.

She continues to have regular visits from friends who love spending time with her, encouraging her to talk and remember events from the past that they have shared with her. They show her endless photos of these happy times together, all helping to rewire her brain; it is invaluable support for someone in her situation and so special that they give time out of their busy days to be with her. She repeats these recollections with them all, as if to try and help herself to remember and reaffirm.

Although Rosie's sleep patterns are markedly improving, she still has a carer with her throughout the night in case she attempts to get out of bed either for the loo or to make her escape. Still unable to stand alone unsupported just yet, the possibility of her falling and banging her head or breaking a limb is too great a risk to take. As well as this night carer, she has a day carer when I am not visiting, who spends time playing simple games with Rosie to try and improve her level of concentration. She is still very vulnerable and totally dependent on those around her so we must put trust in the people who care for her. I try not to jump to conclusions too often as the staff are always very stretched, coping with so many patients in this transitional post traumatic stage of their recovery.

I am home again for my now regular Monday in Dorset. I have become so accustomed to my hospital routine and struggle to be able to get stuck into anything meaningful at home other than catching up on lost sleep and pottering about the house and park in a rather aimless fashion. It's fast approaching the caravan park opening time so there is busyness everywhere. Soon we will have hundreds of caravanning and camping neighbours coming and going for the next seven months. I have appreciated these last months of freedom more than ever on the few occasions I have been here.

When I am here, thoughts of Rosie and what daily progress she may have made are never far from my mind. I churn over the events of each week and mentally record Rosie's progress. I reflect on the two completely separate existences I have at present and struggle to picture in my mind's eye what my old life was like, these memories of the past fading as a new path emerges. I try not to think too hard about what the future will hold for us all and half-heartedly search for distractions to keep my brain from creating any negative storylines and scripts.

My next visit finds a significant improvement in Rosie's voice. She has persevered with the exercises at her speech and language session, and is now sounding very like her old self with her vocal cords now near to normal.

It's wonderful to hear that she has eaten a 'full English', indicating that her appetite is steadily returning to normal; and she is gaining the weight she so desperately needs to get stronger.

It's wonderful to witness these changes in you, my love. How far you have come from your mute and marasmus state in a matter of weeks. To see you gain your strength and to conquer every milestone with such determination is you all over. You never give up, do you? You showed me that when you were younger, that day you clung for your life on that bolting pony as it headed off up the lane and out of sight; despite your inexperience at riding ponies, you hung on. That's your grit, that is, your trademark mettle and grit!

It is hard to pinpoint Rosie's last memory exactly as she is still so amnesic. She has no memory of her accident and we have often wondered if she remembers anything about her work, as she had only been with the company a short while. A few of her work colleagues pay their first visit and she can recognise and name them all. They are encouraged to see the progress she has made. We still can't let our thoughts go too far adrift as we wonder if she will ever be back working with them again; it's evident that the gap that exists at this present time between the possibility and the reality is far too large. We mustn't lose hope for her, though, and must focus on the here and now and the progress she is making.

As the days pass, Rosie is giving us the impression that she can now understand a little more about where she is, although she has no idea how to get from her bed to the day room. If she were able to walk independently, she would perhaps have more practice in orientating herself within the ward. She continues each day with her constant stream of questions and refuses to rest her lively brain for very long. It's hard to explain to her that she needs to rest in order to recover. Rosie's behaviour reminds me of herself as a child, questioning everything and chattering away to her heart's content. This IS her very nature and we must allow her to follow her own pattern of recovery.

Today Lauren and I take Rosie for her regular afternoon tea in the hospital café, always a mission in her wonky wheelie chair negotiating the uneven pathways and many people in the bustling environment. Occasionally we catch a bit of uneven camber underneath a wheel and have visions of her going flying out of her chair, leading us to chuckle and joke about being rescued again by a dashing paramedic.

This noisy and busy café environment can still make Rosie feel irritated and exhausted as her brain struggles to decipher conversation from the background noise. She copes incredibly well, and we are amazed when she asks Lauren if her rent is due. Somewhere there must be a connection with her rent payment being due as it's the end of the month.

We have a significant breakthrough as Rosie retains her first bit of new information. Adrian and the boys attended an Arsenal match the evening before and when quizzed the following morning Rosie remembers exactly where they have been. This must mean her brain is improving and that it is able to lay down new anterograde memories which can be built on over time. It's a key observation for her therapy team, another tick in the box that she needs in order to transition to the rehab unit. We are excited to be told that she will move on the 9th of March to the Wolfson, as a bed has become available.

Chapter 19

Physical Challenges and Tea-making

Rosie and I spend the days chatting around her therapy appointments and playing simple games: Connect Four, Pairs to help her memory, and Snap. She is increasingly more fluent in the use of her phone, accessing the apps with ease and sending Snapchats and simple text messages to the family. This is great practice for her as she can now start to use her phone as an aid for her memory as well as her paper diary. In this modern world, we sometimes curse the constant use of phones and technology, but these can be of such benefit in the recovery of brain injury survivors.

As Rosie improves on her exercise bike and makes progress with her strength and coordination, the staff test her to see if she can remember the simple process of how to make a cup of tea. This can sometimes be a challenge after an injury, often due to the brain's slow processing ability and jumbled thought processes: remembering the sequence, what each item is used for, what to put in first, and having the ability and motor control to judge the flow of water and when to stop it. I accompany her together with her rehabilitation technician to a small kitchen within the hospital wing and I observe with amazement. She sits upon a high stool with the necessary ingredients on the worktop in front of her and starts the process. She needs no prompts and remembers exactly what to do. To watch her complete this task in a way that is remarkably close to her pre-accident self is quite staggering. This is proof that there will be more to come in terms of her long-term memory and physical recovery. It never ceases to excite us all as to what she will do next.

The weekend approaches and we get the go-ahead to branch further afield and plan a shopping trip to Tooting with the whole family. This is something Rosie has certainly encoded into her memory, since it involves shopping.

In preparation for this and, as it's a lovely spring day, Rosie's physio coordinator suggests we do a practice run outside around a small square block of buildings, incorporating as much supported walking as we can to see how she copes. We set off out of the hospital grounds with her for the first time since her admission in November last year; and this feels good for us all. Rosie even manages to name one or two spring flowers along the way. She manages to complete most of the walk on foot, heavily supported on either side by Adrian and her physio, with me behind, following closely with her chair for any breaks she may need. She thoroughly enjoys herself, wobbling as she goes but, as she has pushed herself so hard, the effects in terms of her fatigue are huge.

I am right behind you with your chair, my love, it's ready in case you fall or need to rest. I watch you closely. The effort you need to do this draws everything from your all, every ounce of energy you have in you. Each tiny step is gold medal progress, each wobbly, tentative move you earn entirely, they are yours; and one day, we hope, you will be able to walk again on your own. I am glancing now to the opposite side of the Blackshaw Road as we meander and spot the large tree I kicked so hard during your early days on intensive care, when that dreadful storming was all you had to give. I choke up. You are a miracle of life.

This is a massive task and an entirely different ball game from walking inside the hospital. It leaves Rosie utterly exhausted, not only with the physical effort it takes for her to walk upright but with her attention span being so short and her brain unable to finely filter, she takes in all the busy London sights and sounds around her which sends her brain into sensory overload.

She has achieved a huge amount today and later rests on her bed to recover. As she does so, she receives a visit from a max fax surgeon who has been asked to investigate a small hard spot or possibly a bit of retained stitchwork which has appeared on her scar tissue wound above her right eye. As we surround her bed and observe his careful prodding, we are shocked to see him extract a tiny black screw that has worked its way out from one of the metal plates above her eye socket. It's quite a surreal moment and it doesn't take us long before the jokes about Rosie having a 'screw loose' come thick and fast. This will certainly be one of those stories to tell the grandchildren.

As Rosie's time on the hospital wards is thankfully drawing to a close, Adrian and I are given the opportunity to view Rosie's brain scans. We compare the scan taken on the day of her accident and before her facial surgery to the one taken a few months after her operation. The completely shattered right side of her face has now been expertly rebuilt, with her eye sockets in complete symmetry and her bone structure repaired to near normal. We are shown powerful images of her residual brain damage including the three different haemorrhages to her frontal lobes and are given hope for her potential recovery. We feel that Rosie's face saved her brain from further damage in many ways, acting like a crumple zone, as this took a huge knock from the impact of the car.

With our understanding enhanced and our lifelong gratitude to these wonderfully skilled and dedicated medical teams that have made Rosie's recovery possible to this point reinforced, her next chapter moves positively along the recovery journey. We feel such relief that this long medical phase that has saved her life is behind us and the therapeutic teams can start in earnest to rebuild and reconnect her to face the outside world again.

Ta-ra to the tubes, the trachis, the tension. Move on from the medicine, the max fax, the misery. So long to the sutures, the storming, the silence. Welcome the Wolfson, the whatever's next, the wondering. Make way for Miss Mowbray, this Marvel, this Miracle!

Chapter 20

Tooting Expedition

In glorious sunshine, we kick off our family excursion to Tooting High Street with a picnic in the small park beside the hospital. There is a clear blue sky full of hope above us, and the birdsong and yellow spring-flowered carpets enhance our urban surroundings as we sit. It's a joy to be outside with the whole family at long last. After our lunch, we wheel Rosie through the back streets to Tooting High Street.

We slowly approach the entrance doors to the shop and Rosie, suddenly compelled by determination, starts launching herself from her chair. We grab her before she has the chance to fall and assist her as she makes her almost stage entrance through the store doors. Rosie's brain injury often gives others the impression that she is a bit drunk. Her speech can be erratic and slurred, and she staggers and sways through the entrance doors. Her smart, knee-length black coat covers her tall, frail, willowy figure and her long flowing blonde hair frames her beautiful face which sports her large sunnies. This scene instantly reminds us of the antics of Patsy Stone in *Absolutely Fabulous*.

Rosie's determination to buy some new tops is high up on her list of priorities and her desire to keep up is amazing. On paying for her chosen items, she cannot remember her card pin code, leaving it to her father to pick up the bill. I think it has to be said that this is certainly a critical bit of information that needs to be recollected, as bankruptcy on our part is something best avoided.

As we say goodbye to the family, Adrian, Rosie and I make our way back to St George's. We stop briefly for a cup of tea in the warm sunshine outside the hospital café. It is obvious the day has exhausted her in every way and her repetitive speech continues relentlessly. She chuckles away at a pigeon pecking at a discarded crisp, as ever looking for an opportunity to see the funny things in life; this is so very much part of her character. We leave the hospital, renewed by the success of today and with hope for many more future outings to come.

We feared Rosie would be wiped out the next day, but she is in fine spirits. She is starting to ask us questions about her accident and is able to concentrate for fifteen minutes to watch a *Friends* DVD. It will take a while for these old favourites to be remembered but it's a great start and she manages to deliver to Pollyanna some of the familiar exchanges of dialogue from their favourite sketches. We are told that as well as eating her own lunch she had polished off half of another patient's, making up for lost time and thoroughly enjoying it.

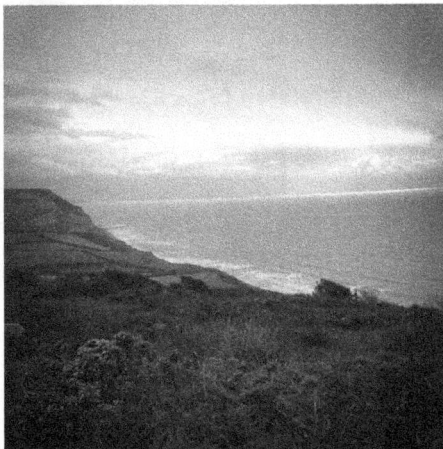

Lovely run on the cliffs this morning before the long
drive back to London! Bye home, see you at
Christmas

Rosie's Instagram post from 3ʳᵈ November 2014:
taken from Stonebarrow Hill, Dorset,
8 days before her accident.

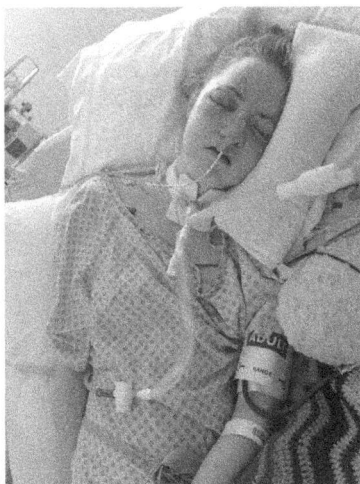

Adrian takes his first photo of Rosie three weeks
after her accident.

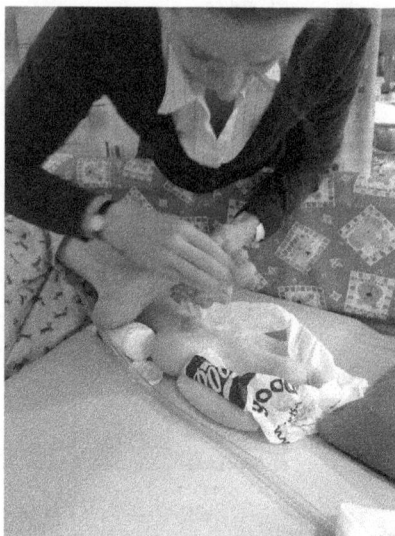

Washing and caring for Rosie's fragile skin and body.

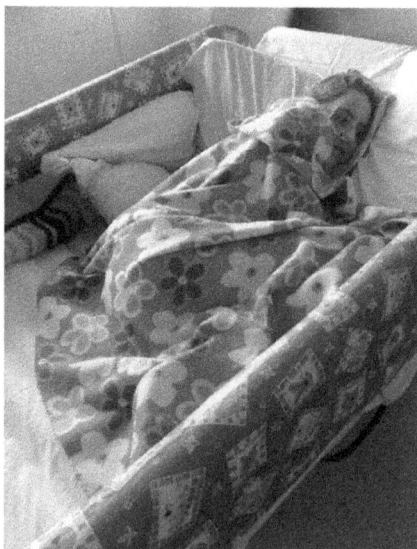

Rosie staring blankly at her bedside protectors.

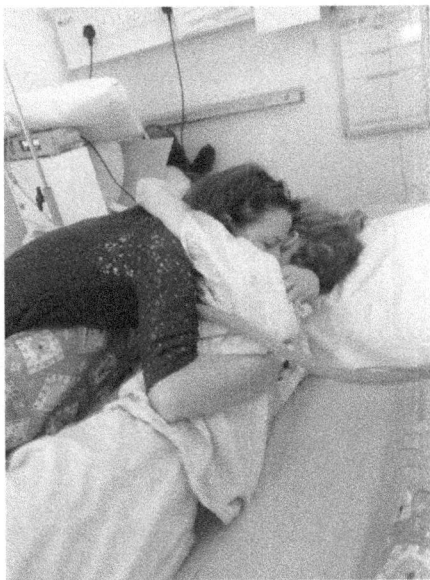

*Christmas Day
'unaware mum hug'.*

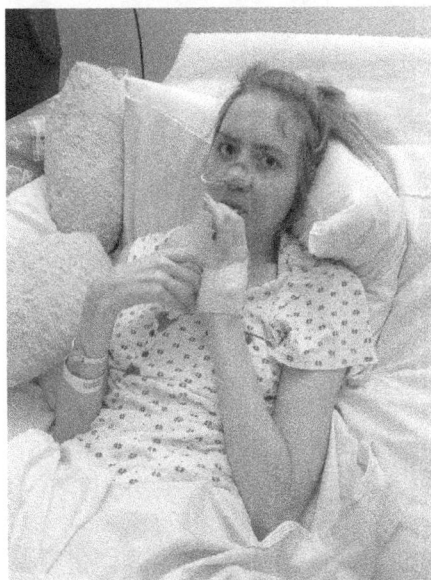

*Rosie drinking
through a straw a
few days before she
started talking.*

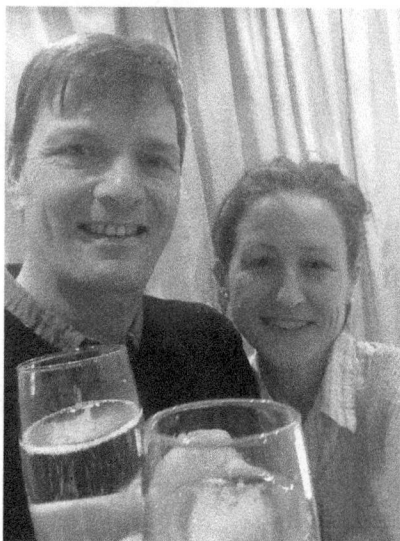

*Celebrating the day
Rosie started
talking again:
January 23rd, 2015.*

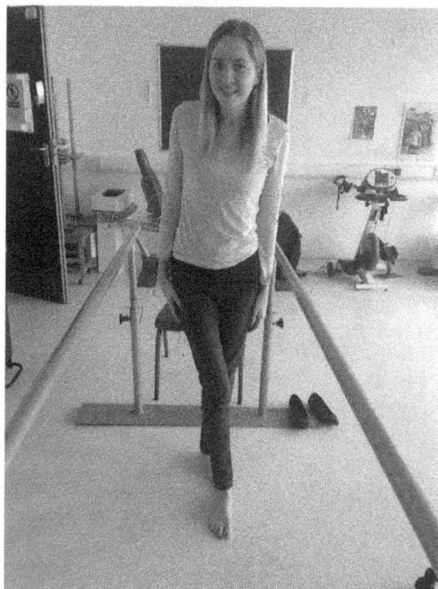

*Learning to balance
and walk again.*

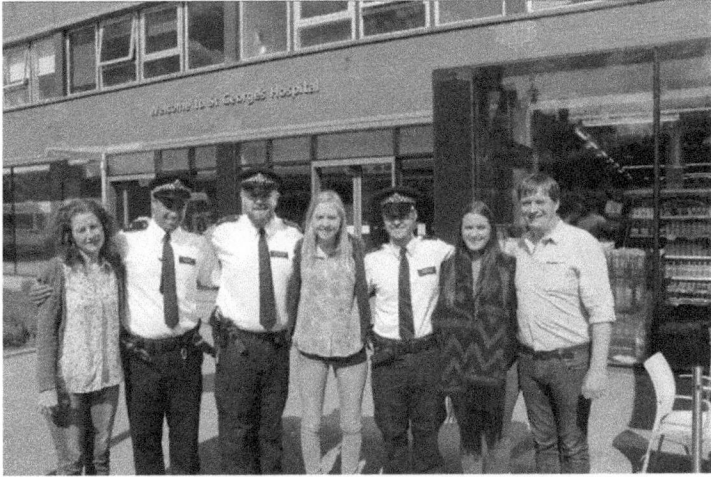

*Meeting and thanking the Met police outside
St George's.*

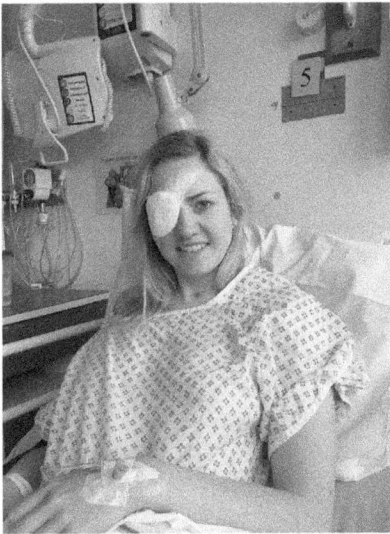

Rosie's eye operation following her discharge to Dorset.

P... is for positivity
March 2015 – April 2016

Chapter 21

Wolfson – Here We Come!

It's a long road up to recovery from here,
A long way back to the light.
A long road up to recovery from here,
A long way to makin' it right.

'Recovery' – Frank Turner

The day has come for Rosie's move to the Wolfson Rehabilitation unit and I arrive to find her all packed up and ready for the off.

The nurses and I trundle Rosie with her bedding and belongings through the many corridors to the opposite side of the hospital and onto the Wolfson unit. We can barely see her face amid the piles of stuff balanced on top of her. We laugh and chat as we go. It's been sad to say goodbye to all the staff on Kent Ward who have seen her through this huge transitional stage of her recovery, but they are all delighted for her to be moving on to rehab.

We settle her into her new bedroom alongside three other patients, filling her surrounding bed area with familiar things to make her feel comfortable. The day continues with a variety of assessments to try and ascertain just how far Rosie has progressed through her very long period of Post Traumatic Amnesia.

She is asked to remember three things and repeat them after half an hour, but sadly she can't manage this. The main patient assessment consists of a set of twelve simple and basic questions, including, for example, her name, the date, month and year, where she is, what's happened to her. These all need to be answered correctly for three consecutive days. When successfully completed, this can confirm a patient is out of their Post Traumatic Amnesia stage. Rosie is unable to pass this test, so it will need to be continued day after day until she can. So far, we are unable to pinpoint Rosie's last memory before her accident and nothing is remembered of the days and weeks leading up it.

She has pockets of retrograde memory. Rosie can remember and visually place her work friends who she had only worked with for a few months before her accident but can't remember any details of the job she used to do with them. She remembers the address of her flat in Merton Road but can't tell us what it looks like or anything about the surrounding area.

These two scenarios clash on the visual right side of her brain and the procedural left, revealing that both are still working together in some slightly haphazard fashion. Her memory for the people in her life seems to be relatively intact. It's difficult to ascertain what new information she has encoded into her deeper memory and what is happening in her more transient working memory. She also struggles with understanding what's happened to her and, at times, thinks she has fallen off a horse. It's as if we are waiting for a huge chunk of memory to return to her. We constantly keep the conversation going in the hope that this might be triggered.

We realise now that the patient boundaries are different in the Wolfson. We are permitted to take Rosie out and about in the car, so Adrian and I decide to take her on a small excursion to the local shopping centre in Colliers Wood. We take her chair but aim to encourage her to walk with our support as much as she can.

It's Will's twenty-first birthday in a week's time so we encourage her to choose a present for him. She purchases a couple of T-shirts from a retail store and pays with her card, remembering her pin code this time (a surprising relief!). We have coffee and lunch out and Rosie chooses exactly the food and drink she would normally have had, thoroughly enjoying her first dining out experience since her accident. We take a detour on our way back to the hospital and pass her flat and the Southfields tube station where she used to catch the train to work but nothing at all is recognised. Passing through the junction where she was knocked down triggers no memory, nor does driving along her usual running route on Durnsford Road. She had done this countless times before her accident.

How do you not remember this, any of it? You used to call me on your way home from work for a chat as you walked back to your flat; I know you knew these roads and shops and pathways. Has nature blotted these memories out completely to shield you from all this trauma and suffering, my love? Does it want to protect you from the very thing that nearly took your life away?

It's mid-March and Mother's Day – a very significant Mother's Day for me this one, as I am very fortunate to still have all my four children. I have decided to come home early from London as I have been struggling with a nasty bronchial infection for some time now. The constant comings and goings to and from the hospital have left me susceptible to this and, not wanting it to be passed to Rosie, I have come home for a few days of rest and recuperation. The thought of Rosie getting yet another infection, particularly as she has been infection-free for some time now, is unbearable.

With Pollyanna, Will and Greg joining us at home, we decide to Facetime Rosie from the kitchen table. She is in good spirits, although constantly wishing she was home. After our car trip confirmed her lack of recognition for some of the familiar places in her life, we have been concerned that she perhaps wouldn't recognise even her familiar, family home. We decide to take the iPad from room to room, asking her if she recognises any of the surroundings and the history of specific objects and pictures and, although some bits are sketchy, she reassures us that her memory for home has been retained.

Once Rosie starts to settle into the Wolfson, she will be having a much more structured day with her therapy sessions, although maybe not as many as she would like. Rosie will be set mutually agreed goals, both short and long term, to work towards as part of her recovery. Her days will start with personal grooming sessions, relearning to do these daily essential routines independently without prompting. She has no trouble in recalling her makeup and hair straightening routine, which doesn't really surprise us too much as it was so ingrained before her accident.

She will have breakfast and lunch in between her therapy sessions in a large dining room alongside all the other patients. There is a day room with TV and a few games should she wish to spend time there. She is issued with a weekly printed timetable to help her get into a regular daily pattern of events. She repeats the contents over and over to herself, trying so hard to retain even the tiniest detail to remember what she is doing and when. She is incredibly muddled most of the time but we hope that in time she will have more ordered thought processes.

It becomes increasingly hard when I leave after my visits, as all she wants to do is come home; but she has yet to show any real sadness at her situation or any emotion other than a little frustration and mostly happiness. It's as if her normal emotional responses are confused or delayed. I guess this makes things a little easier for us in some ways, as to leave her distraught would be very painful. She does cooperate well with her therapists and continues to push herself at each session.

Chapter 22

Weekends Out

We are now able to take Rosie out and about each weekend and plan a birthday lunch in Tooting with the family to celebrate Will's 21st birthday – our first proper family lunch out, which proves a lovely one: birthday cake, presents and laughter. After lunch Rosie asks if she can go back to her flat for the afternoon. On arrival, she eagerly attempts to scale the steep steps to the front door, closely guarded by us following behind. She enjoys checking her clothes wardrobe and her baking cupboard. With her memory so vague, it's sometimes hard to gauge if she really remembers much about her time spent here with Lauren. I can see that this is truly difficult for Lauren to get to grips with, as this is not the Rosie she remembers.

Bringing her back here is a stark reminder for all of us that this is going to be a long, long process; and the following day reaffirms our worries when Rosie is unable to remember even visiting her flat the day before, or many of the details within it.

We have been informed that a lot of the patients can leave the Wolfson at weekends if they are able to and this is greatly encouraged. We decide to make enquires as to how to prepare for this.

On weekdays I often have lunch with Rosie and eat my sandwiches with her just to support her a little into this new phase. As often as I can, I take her outside in her chair to the little park next to St George's during her free timetable periods. This alleviates her boredom and the change of air and scenery perks her up. Otherwise, she sits alone in her room for long periods in between therapies. Her carer is there to offer help with her orientation and memory through conversation and games and assists her to other areas of the centre as she can't navigate herself just yet. She is unable to confidently walk unaided for more than a short period of time and still needs support with this to mitigate the risk of falling.

One of her work colleagues has lent her an iPad and has kindly installed some useful brain improvement game apps for her to use. She begins her own initiated daily timetable of practice, the start of a regular and long-lasting pattern of relearning that has proved invaluable to her brain's recovery.

The Wolfson team hold regular family meetings, which Adrian and I attend, to update us on Rosie's progress. They help set her new goals to work towards. She has expressed for some time that she would like to stay at her flat some weekends and visit her home in Dorset for Easter and her birthday. We are given the OK for both.

We will start with a night away in her flat, providing it is suitable enough to accommodate her physical challenges and is safe. Once her Occupational Therapist has paid a visit and the necessary boxes have been ticked, this can go ahead. The OT arranges a meeting with me at the flat to identify any obstacles and danger points to look out for and I must always sleep next to her in case she falls out of bed. We are all excited, if a little apprehensive, about the weekend stay but will take it at Rosie's pace, which will no doubt be faster than ours.

Rosie is up, ready and waiting for us to take her to her flat when we arrive to collect her. After settling in she seems a little more familiar with the surroundings than the last time we visited so some memories must have been stimulated somewhere. It's a beautiful day so we decide to wheel her through King George's Park and to Southside shopping centre for lunch and a bit of retail therapy; this never fails to keep her spirits high. Apart from running, shopping is her next favourite pastime. We tentatively push her in her chair through the shopping centre, a real skill that needs to be practised when you have had limited experience of negotiating a wheelchair in busy places. To our surprise, a nurse who looked after Rosie on Brodie Ward stops us to chat. She is amazed to see how far Rosie has improved from those early days when she was very poorly.

We pop into Rosie's favourite shop for undies and the supermarket to collect some food items for a Sunday roast we plan to cook tomorrow. The afternoon is spent enjoying tea, cake and a board game and in the evening, we have a Chinese takeaway and a glass or two of wine, all of which are washed down with the usual Saturday night telly. This all seems quite surreal at times and, with Rosie constantly chatting and retaining tiny bits of information as we answer her wide range of questions, we feel as though improvements are gradually starting to happen.

I sleep with Rosie that night and ponder on the last time she slept here and the chain of events since then. It must feel very daunting for her to be here after so long: such a contrast to the last four and half months in St George's Hospital.

You stir at times in your sleep and sit bolt upright; I reassure you and you settle back down. It must seem strange for you to be back here again, my love. I too have sat bolt upright here, in this bed, during my restless sleep, in battle with my anxious nightmares about you and for you. We lie now side by side and I watch you; I hear your gentle breathing, I sense your subtle movements as you slumber, and I weep a little. My tears are for something different now: they are for gratitude, for that unique mother and child love that is still alive today, for us; a bond that carries such a power that cannot be explained, only felt in the depths of my beating heart.

In the morning, as we prepare our roast lunch, Rosie voices her concern about being out of the hospital; she feels, perhaps, that we have taken her away of our own accord. This, we come to understand over time, is the effect of her institutionalisation from being in hospital for so long. We have work to do to reassure her, and it might take a while for her to feel comfortable with these new freedoms she will be given. We all agree it has been a thoroughly successful first overnight trip as we return her to the Wolfson for the start of another week.

We are informed that during mid-April, the Wolfson will be relocating its more able patients to a brand-new centre based at Queen Mary's Hospital in Roehampton; and as long as her memory and her physical challenges improve further, Rosie should be able to continue her rehabilitation there until she is ready to leave permanently. We do a recce of Queen Mary's while we have the chance and it's a much lighter, more spacious environment than St George's and has been purpose built for a wide variety of rehabilitation needs.

As Rosie settles into her weekly pattern, I now need to adjust mine too and I plan to spend my weekdays back home in Dorset from now on. Adrian and I will come back up on a Friday, take Rosie out for the weekend and return her back to the Wolfson on Sunday afternoon. We envisage taking her home to Dorset or to her flat each weekend for the remainder of her stay in hospital. This will take some getting used to for us but we embrace the change and try not to think too hard about the eight-hour Dorset to London turnaround twice each weekend if she comes home. It will be worth the effort as she will come back here after she leaves hospital to continue her rehabilitation with us in Dorset.

Chapter 23

Dorset for Easter

Easter is looming fast and we start planning the long weekend at home with much excitement mixed with anxiety. I run through, with the nurse in charge of arrangements, how we are going to accomplish the challenges of the stairs, showering, Rosie's sleeping arrangements and her fatigue, unaware that the first tricky problem would be the car journey home.

The Easter traffic is heavy and congested as we travel down and Rosie and Pollyanna ease the tedium by singing along to various songs. When Rosie was in hospital, towards the end of her Post Traumatic Amnesia stage, she could remember almost word for word the song lyrics from one of her favourite artists, Frank Turner, but couldn't remember what she had eaten minutes beforehand. We never cease to be amazed by her brain's functioning – always blowing us away with her memory for the music she enjoys.

As we join the notoriously bad A31, we get into a jam and the car's stop and start motion, together with Rosie's constant flicking through her phone, makes her feel very nauseous. We manage to catch her just in time as we swing off the road onto a verge. Car travel motion will take a bit of getting used to now that she has a very different tolerance to movement due to her brain injury.

We arrive home and Rosie immediately starts familiarising herself. Over the weekend, as her energy and memory permit, she settles, sleeping well with either myself or Pollyanna beside her and managing to take a few more steps unaided. Perhaps it's being somewhere she knows that helps.

Over the weekend we have visits from family and friends who all help to evoke Rosie's memories and encourage her into conversation. This is so vitally important for many reasons to help her brain rewire and for her to feel part of what's happening. She keeps up well and switches off when she needs to, although her switching off is an iPad full of brain games, rather than the regular nap which we continually try to encourage.

The weekend is taken very slowly as Rosie is still very fragile and tentative about walking and is very vague a lot of the time. We are always on high alert for obstacles she could trip over and situations that she might find overwhelming. Her spirits are high, though, and her humour continues to bring back to us elements of the girl we all know.

We all feel relieved to be back: the first time at home together in months. We are complete now that Monty is back home in his favourite place, licking the dirty dishes and cutlery as we stack the dishwasher each evening and filling the house with those smells only a dog can produce. We play Jenga and introduce Rosie to Dobble – a game that has become a firm family favourite after Greg introduced it to lift our spirits on evenings after many a weary hospital visit. We make a visit to the local supermarket and on Saturday evening we have a takeaway.

Having my family home again after so many difficult months is such a relief, and so comforting; and I find myself doing a double take sometimes when I hear Rosie fully engaged in the laughter and quick-fire exchanges of conversation as we eat our Easter Sunday roast – it could all have been so very different.

Do you remember the little nests of eggs I made for you all every Easter? I would use hay from the shed and picked moss and twigs from the wood next to our house on the farm. I would sneak them beside your beds before the dawn of Easter day. And the Foot and Mouth Disease outbreak? Do you remember that dreadful Easter of confinement, the stench of the rotting carcasses from the barn next door, the sight of burning pyres of animals from all the farms in the valley? You all hung over the shed door, your hands full with little bunches of spring flowers, throwing them onto your pet lambs and saying goodbye to them as they lay still, waiting to join those pyres. We have all grown beyond the years from that sad time, haven't we, and I know we shall grow from this time too.

As we all start the long haul back up to London in convoy, we immediately encounter a diversion through the country lanes. A thatched pub in the local village has caught fire and the main road has had to be closed. With a caravan jack-knifed in front of our traffic queue, Adrian and Edd leave our cars to offer assistance. The constant stopping and starting and jerks from the car combined with the unexpected heat of the spring sun make Rosie feel very nauseous.

We get out of the car, Rosie in her stockinged feet. Pollyanna, Dani and I assist her with her sickness; and when we turn around, we observe the traffic is on the move again and Adrian and Edd are now driving their cars away from us all. With Rosie unable to walk any real distance and without shoes, I promptly heave her on to my back and start to jog cautiously back to the car which is now stationary again. This bizarre scene of me piggy-backing my injured, sickly adult daughter past cars full of bad-tempered holidaymakers makes us all giggle, bringing release to a potentially stressful situation. Thankfully, the rest of the journey proceeds without a hitch.

As the weeks continue, Rosie's timetable gradually gets busier. Physiotherapy sessions work on her core strength, stability and confidence with walking; psychology helps her to develop her insight into what's happened to her; and speech and language therapy aims to expand her memory connections and language using very simple cards. Some of these cards depict familiar everyday objects, such as an iron or a utensil, and others everyday situations: for example, a person eating, driving or cooking. There are small conversation groups added to the mix which help to promote language.

Rosie has started using an app called 'One Day' which aims to assist her memory, using photos of her participating in activities with added text to prompt her, all with the aim of building up a pattern for her to increase her retention and recall. She still has regular visits from friends who report progress to us and, with gaps in our visits too, we notice these improvements. Although this progress is not quite as fast as we had hoped, we are now slowly understanding that the timescale for recovery from severe brain injury is not in terms of weeks or months, but in years and years.

I try not to dwell on our future too much at this stage, my love. It's so hard sometimes, hard not to jump to the years ahead of us, to scenarios that may or may not happen and conclusions that could all be so wrong. We must live in the moments of each phase of your recovery that remain with the ebb and the flow of the passing of time.

Chapter 24

Adrian's 50th and the Rude Aussie

Adrian's 50th birthday falls on Rosie's last weekend at the Wolfson, St George's and before her transfer to the new Wolfson at Queen Mary's Hospital in Roehampton. It just so happens that Arsenal, the family's favourite footie team, are playing in the FA cup semi-final at Wembley; so we arrange the day around a pub outing to watch the game followed by a meal out at The Castle pub in Tooting. Rosie looks stunning, wearing her graduation dress again for the occasion. We are excited for the day ahead of us.

When we are out and about amongst the crowds, we are becoming more aware of how other people view Rosie. For the moment, she is largely unaware of the stares from others, but we notice this behaviour on a regular basis. People actually stop in their tracks, turning their heads and intently gawping at her up and down. Not knowing quite how to cope with this new situation ourselves, we feel quite defensive at times and have become quite accustomed to catching them out by making eye contact and giving them a hard stare back. Sometimes I'm not sure if people even realise they are doing this; but they do get the message when we ask them politely but firmly not to stare. I often wonder what they think. Is it because Rosie is tall, blonde, slim and beautiful? Or are they just wondering what her story is, when they see her limping, awkward gait, and her stilted, slow movements?

After the match, we leave the noisy pub with Rosie ahead of me. As we exit, I am distracted by an Australian man who catches my arm to stop me. "What's wrong with that girl?" he asks in a beer-fuelled slur.

"That girl happens to be my daughter and she has had an accident," I state firmly as I walk off, asking myself why he said what he did: is he just being nosy? Has his family been affected by that curveball? Has he a sister who looks similar? Is he a medical student inquisitive for his dissertation? Or just a very rude man? – I shall never know the answer, but this all gives us an idea of what to expect over time. We must develop a thicker layer of skin and ignore as much as we can the disdainful behaviour of some others.

We move swiftly on – after tutting and hissing at this incident – to a wonderful celebratory meal. It has been Adrian's wish, his one and only longed-for birthday present, to have Rosie join him for his birthday meal; and this has happened just the way he wanted, together with the rest of the family, marking this milestone birthday in the most memorable of ways.

Chapter 25

Queen Mary's – the Last Leg

Leaving St George's today has been very emotional. This amazing hospital and its wonderful and dedicated staff have saved the life of our daughter and brought her back to us. As we visit the wards in turn to say our goodbyes and offer thanks, everyone is delighted to see Rosie again; and their encouraging remarks on her progress warm our hearts.

Rosie will now spend the last five weeks of her long rehabilitation stint at Queen Mary's. Her therapy sessions will continue with many of the same staff from St George's. After settling her into her new room and briefly acquainting ourselves with the new staff, we leave her in the day room with other inpatients for company and head back to Dorset to prepare for her homecoming next weekend to celebrate her own birthday.

My new routine at home has taken a bit of getting used to over these last weeks but I am enjoying my days of freedom, taking walks on the cliffs with Monty, and having the odd cup of tea with a friend.

I frequently walk around the garden; the withering spring flowers are now making way for the appearance of summer's spectacle and the trees are now laden with green lusciousness. I lean over the wonky fence that surrounds my neglected veg patch and view, with some sadness, last autumn's unworked soil full of clods and weeds, and the greenhouse, unkempt and empty. I dig deep to drum up some enthusiasm but, as it's nearly the end of April, I have missed most of this season's greenhouse sowing and planting. Thinking now about the near future, I'm unclear of what to expect when Rosie comes home; so, I make a pact with myself to give 'all things veg-growing' a miss for this year, the first time for many years. It's a hard but necessary decision.

That's where you could always guarantee to find me, in my veg patch. "Can I eat a tomato / pick a cucumber or some beans?" "What's for supper?" You have watched me over the years, my love, inside my earthy bubble. I loved that feeling, pottering in the late afternoon sun, collecting the garden produce in my old willow basket to add to our suppers. The thrill of seeing the abundance and the disappointment when discovering the scarcity when scavenged by the garden's wildlife was all part of it; each year was something new. I must leave this time for now and return to it later…

Rosie texts me frequently from the hospital. Her days are filled with therapies and she texts me in brief what she has done, using her diary as her reference. She is still unable to retain much new information in any quantity, but we see little increments of progress.

We arrive at her bedside to collect her for her birthday weekend home. Her bags are packed and ready, but there is no sign of Rosie.

Standing beside her bed is a sweet elderly lady with a bible in hand. She is unsure exactly where Rosie is but rather enthusiastically announces that Rosie has signed up for the Christian evening course that takes place at the hospital. Adrian and I reply, our wry smiles a bit of a giveaway.

"We're not sure if Rosie quite understands what she is doing at the moment. We feel fairly sure she would not sign up as she has always, and often quite profoundly, protested her atheist beliefs." The woman rather apologetically suggests that perhaps Rosie isn't quite the patient she was looking for and maybe it was someone else in the next room.

When Rosie eventually returns with her carer she laughs, true to form, and tells us that no, she hasn't been converted, despite her brain injury.

Chapter 26

Rosie's Birthday Shenanigans

We reach another of Rosie's goals, her birthday weekend at home.

All the family are coming back to celebrate. It's a good feeling now that we are all able to regroup at home in Dorset in a familiar relaxed environment, rather than being cooped up by a hospital bedside or in a cramped day room.

We hit the Dorset home road yet again. Rosie is now coping much better with the journey, largely due to the travel tablets which keep her sickness at bay.

As the journey progresses, she announces that she is desperate for the loo. Normally, I am the one who needs the loo at regular intervals. Eagerly trying to find the next convenient service station but to no avail, we have no choice but to swing on to the verge at the next roundabout. Fortunately a small gate leads to a discreet area suitable for emptying a bursting bladder.

We help Rosie out of the car, but we hadn't quite thought through our plan of execution beforehand. Rosie can barely stand alone for long, let alone crouch down in a squatting position and hold herself there for the duration. We suggest to Rosie that we assist her in much the same way as we did when she was a child. She laughs at the memory of her childhood 'wee lifts' in outdoor spaces, getting stingers on the bottom in the process. We respect her reluctance at finding herself in this unusual situation now that she is an adult, but we all agree that we are left with no choice when "a girl's got to do what a girl's got to do." So, with Adrian one side of her and myself the other, lifting each of her legs whilst suggesting to Rosie that she "get a move on" as our backs are not going to hold out for too much longer, we wait; and as we do, she gets a fit of the giggles, and before long we find ourselves in a comical, messy heap on the ground, with the mission unaccomplished. After composing ourselves, and following one or two further attempts, we are – thankfully – successful; so we continue our journey joking and laughing about the events that have just occurred and under normal circumstances confirm that … THAT would NOT have happened!

Rosie's weekend is an enjoyable one all round. We take her swimming in the caravan park pool; she manages a short spurt of doggy paddle but is visibly exhausted afterwards. It's going to be some time before she swims like the fish she once was.

The following weekend we repeat the same journey home (minus the loo stop), this time with Lauren; and we have another enjoyable weekend away from the city. We attempt a walk on the cliffs, Rosie managing some steep steps with our aid and not giving up on her challenges.

We repeat these home routines until she leaves hospital. It's an arduous weekend of travel but worth it to have these few precious hours at home and it helps Rosie acclimatise to the home environment she will be in for a considerable period of convalescence and healing once she leaves hospital.

We eat on the hoof, as we have done so often recently, regular mealtimes now a thing of the past. I never imagined that I would have to visit an infamous burger outlet again, at least not before any grandchildren come along and badger me to take them (somewhat reluctantly) there; but for now they fill the gap when you are famished and out of energy and ideas for supper.

Rosie still repeats herself much of the time but her conversation is improving and, although she still gives the impression she has 'had a few', her speech is making improvements too. She is yet to show any real emotion other than happiness and frustration. Rosie has always been an 'April shower', but largely on the sunny side of this. I have a theory that when she was hit, her endorphins and her sense of well-being must have been at their highest because of her run, so that maybe this has left her with the more upbeat, happier elements of her personality rather than feelings of low mood. We'll have to wait to see.

I long for you to cry, my love, for you to visibly show us what you are feeling deep within your soul. I need you to demonstrate those emotions; I can comfort you then, in the way that I know how. Have these feelings been stunned and frozen in your being? You laugh the way you did, and anger the way you did; but what about your sorrow? Surely you must feel such sadness for your state? But self-pity was never really you. Your tender heart would often touch upon the sorry states of others. "Mummy, can I raise money for the

Kosovan refugees?" Your coffee morning was a great success; and as for your abseil for NSPCC, that took some nerve, didn't it? I yearn for even a fragment of this emotion to return to you.

Chapter 27

Polling Day Pride

On weekdays, Rosie continues with her full timetable. This week she has an outside task set for her. It incorporates a trip on the bus to Putney and shopping for ingredients to make a simple meal, all guided by her occupational therapists and physios as they encourage her to take the lead in finding a coffee shop via Google and the local supermarket. These are the very first steps to independence and it is clear to us all at this moment that Rosie will need time and support once she comes home before she is able to carry out tasks independently and without risk. She completes this supported challenge and copes well, despite the challenging weather conditions. Even something as subtle as a gentle breeze as she walks can disorientate her as her brain has to work hard to cope with the many sensory distractions of the busy city environment. She still can't walk a great distance unaided, so her focus is very much down towards the pavement and not on her surroundings, which can be hazardous.

As the build-up for the general election reaches its finale on May 7th, Rosie is determined to have her say. We have always encouraged our children to vote and consider it a privilege to live in a democratic society. We set off to Southfields from the hospital and Rosie, as determined as ever, walks into the station, polling card in hand and, with a little assistance, casts her vote stating,

"If I can do this then there is no excuse for anyone else," and we totally agree, feeling immensely proud of her for exercising her right.

The following week we take a trip with Rosie into her old workplace: her first tube ride for months. Her work friends have been so supportive and everyone is keen to see her return to her desk. She chats away, making friendly conversation with her colleagues, remembering most of them; but she has absolutely no recollection as to what she did in her job role, even though she sat at her own desk while she was there. It's as if this whole section of her memory has been either wiped out or is not yet ready to return.

We so hope over time that these detailed memories will return as she makes improvements and that she will be able to continue up the career ladder she had planned.

As we say our goodbyes to her back at the hospital, we notice a sudden drop in her mood and she pleads with us to take her home as the tears start to fall. It's hard to say that you are happy when someone cries but, through our comforting and consoling and tears of our own, we are relieved to see this change in her mood from the fairly blunt-edged but cheerful disposition since her emergence from PTA.

You cried today and revealed to us your fragility, your tentative connection to the baring of your deeper self, and I cried too. The significance of witnessing you feel again is incalculable; this offers you an opening now to connect with yourself again in time, a starting point to the self, the awareness, the confidence and the worth.

We explain Rosie's evident sadness to her team, and they all feel that she would make more progress at home with us now, supported by community rehabilitation. The wheels are duly put into motion for her transfer from hospital rehab to the community brain injury rehab team in Dorset. Once the necessary paperwork has been completed and the multi-disciplinary team in Dorset are on board, we can prepare for Rosie's transfer home.

Chapter 28

Leaving Hospital for Dorset

So open the shutters, raise up the mast,
rejoice, rebuild, the storm has passed.
Cast off the crutches, cut off the cast,
rejoice, rebuild, the storm has passed.

'The Next Storm' – Frank Turner.

After nearly six and a half months in hospital and rehab, the date has now arrived for Rosie to leave the Wolfson for good. Friday 22nd May 2015 will always be a day we remember. It really is monumental for all of us and we never really envisaged it would happen. We have our final family meeting, dictating the way forward in terms of care and support, and say our heartfelt goodbyes to all the team who have continued supporting Rosie throughout this final stage of her confinement. Her lovely psychologist's parting words to us are, "One day you, as a family, may come to appreciate everything in your lives in a different way than you did before this happened. I have found many families do." I shall bear this in mind as we move on to the next stages of Rosie's recovery. As we leave, we vow to be back to visit when time allows.

As we drive away from Queen Mary's for the last time, my mind starts to contemplate the prospect of what happens now. I have been advised that the Dorset brain injury team will make contact with me over the next few weeks to arrange visits and assessments for Rosie and discuss the way forward with Rosie and myself from here.

I think about how this might have been, the countless unknowns we could have faced at this point of time. During the early days, many times in my head I had reorganised a downstairs room to cope with a bedridden, fully dependent daughter with no prospects of recovery. I wonder how we would have managed in the long term had we been given this burden of responsibility. There is no question that we are facing a difficult set of challenges now, but nothing to what potentially could have been. Many other families contend with far worse and we must remind ourselves to count our blessings on a daily basis, however tough it may get.

As we settle back at home and I start caring for Rosie, it's not long before I experience a huge wave of fear and anxiety as reality hits me. All through these past months, Rosie's routines have been safely and firmly in control of the hospital and, as time has gone on, my own daily pattern of independence here at home has been reinstated to a degree. Now, I am met with a completely contrasting set of boundaries.

I suppose we have never consciously had any vision of what the future would look like for each of our children. We have always encouraged them to do what makes them happy. I have seen too many disillusioned students and pushy parents during my years working in a busy secondary school reception. Encouraging our children to go with their hearts has always been top of the list for

Adrian and me. Sometimes I was so caught up with work myself and our busy everyday lives that there was no time to contemplate what their futures would hold.

Adrian and I had a 1970s comprehensive school and college education so hadn't really considered university as a path for our children but they all chose to take this route and have never looked back. They all had completely different subjects of study and work interests, which has made life so interesting.

As the university years came upon us, I started to get used to the fact that the children would now move further afield and create their own lives. Life and the opportunities it had to offer would be unlocked for them all. Although our closeness has always been pretty steadfast, living in each other pockets was not something any of us would have wanted. Adrian and I have felt incredibly proud of our offspring and their achievements. As hard as it was to have them living some distance away, the metaphorical umbilical cord had to adjust, and I had to adjust with it.

I found myself free to do as I pleased with no dependent children at home. I worked part-time and enjoyed my leisure time. Adrian and I got used to having our own space; we could go away as and when work allowed with no responsibilities other than the dog and cat. I am now starkly faced for the foreseeable future with supporting a dependent adult daughter who I can't leave alone, or at least not for the time being. Nothing and no one has prepared me for this. Life will now change, and I feel unexpectedly as if I am reversing at speed, thrown back in years to some sort of time warp.

The only skill set I have is my experience of motherhood and a reasonable quota of practical and emotional intelligence. It feels a very scary place to be at times and I feel sure it will take some time to adjust to this new role. The one thing I am totally convinced of deep down in my heart is that, however robbed I feel of my own independence, I will not give up on my daughter's recovery; she will be my main priority for as long as it takes – her life is so infinitely changed, in ways far beyond the changes to my own.

Over the following weeks, being at home and in a more relaxed setting, Rosie increasingly develops her own routine with me assisting as her needs dictate. We sit each morning over breakfast and she repeats the same things regularly until they start to be retained: "How old is the cat?" and "When did we get her?" "Who are my relations?" and "How do they fit into the family?" "How long have we lived here?" She also asks about family holidays and her life before her accident. All her repeated questions are very important and fundamental, facts that have to be relearned. They prompt memories that are attached to them, mapping her mind to painstakingly build up the layers of her life before her accident. It's as if her brain has to kickstart its new pathways and by doing this, it is firing up the neurons linking information together which, as she improves, will be vital to her memory retention and cognitive improvement. We continue with this tirelessly and move at her pace of convalescence, the home environment being the support blanket she needs for this to happen.

Bear with me, my love, as I bear with you. I know we won't get it right all the time; we are all learning together on this journey. This is now the true start of your homeward path to come back to us, to rebuild yourself back to you, the pieces of this broken jigsaw slotting together, a few frayed edges; that's what we all have, isn't it, frayed edges. That's what makes us human and who we are, our imperfections more perfect than we give them credit for.

Family life continues alongside Rosie's recovery, with its highs as well as the lows. Our high at the moment is the announcement of Edd and Dani's engagement, with their wedding planned for July next year; and we are all uplifted at this news. Edd was hoping to propose to Dani while they were in Sweden last Christmas but, as Rosie was still in her unaware state and so poorly, he felt that she would be really upset and confused if she had woken up to find that that had happened during her minimal conscious state. How wonderful that she is awake and can digest and retain this fantastic news: real evidence that some new information is staying with her.

As the start of the preparations begin, we feel excited about the prospect of Rosie being a bridesmaid and walking up the aisle behind Dani. It's some time away but Rosie has certainly been assigned a new goal, to work hard to improve at her walking.

Chapter 29

Ants in my Brain… and Weetabix Have Feelings

I encourage Rosie regularly to make her own breakfast and to improve on her domestic capabilities and she is gradually getting more familiar with where things are kept in the kitchen, although prompting is helpful. This is an ongoing task for her as her memory is still very vague and virtually non-existent at times. She struggles to remember anything she did yesterday but frequently makes light of her situation.

One morning, while Rosie is in the kitchen making her breakfast and I am in the next room, a high pitched "Oh no!" resonates through the air from her direction. I hot-foot it in to see what's happened and ask her, as she pours milk onto her Weetabix, what the matter is. And this is her reply: "It's the Weetabix. I think they are saying, 'Oh no, that's too cold' as I pour this milk on them. I'm sure Weetabix must have feelings." I am tickled by her comments and warmed by the evident compassionate side of her personality making its appearance again.

We laugh, as I ask her, "What does it actually feel like in your brain?"

"It feels like I have loads of ants milling about inside my head," she replies. With this, Rosie affirms my ant analogy and it's in this exact moment that the title of my book was born.

You captivated me today with your sensitivity, your gentle kindness, even though it was only the Weetabix you expressed those feelings towards. What I witnessed today, my love, I feel will be translated to human feeling. You have shown that's not been lost, that you still feel the empathy you always had. And the ants: well, I can't explain that for you at this stage other than that those neurons are doing their hard work.

Chapter 30

Rehab Repetition!

Over the following weeks after Rosie leaves hospital, we start to have regular daily visits from the community brain injury team, continuing the long pattern of therapies to help her improve further.

Her occupational therapist works her through domestic chores, goal-setting and physiotherapy exercises to help mobilise her more and improve her balance and flexibility. Rosie's main goal now after being at home for a while is to get back to London and work again. Her neuro psychologist helps her with insight following her accident: we often hear the term 'lack of insight' frequently used in brain injury recovery, and I often got the impression in the early days that this is something that should happen instantly, that Rosie should suddenly accept everything that's happened to her in one fell swoop. It doesn't happen like that. How can a person possibly understand their situation, and the effect it has had, particularly when they are so far removed from their previous life? It takes years. Insight and acceptance run alongside the person as they live and grow after their injury; and working closely with a neuro psychologist is key to achieving this successfully.

Rosie's Speech and Language therapist sets tasks to improve her memory and language skills, continuing along the same lines as the Wolfson. She is asked to remember a string of words whilst being completely distracted for some time on another task, then asked to recall them. She has a brain injury workbook of exercises and small written and verbal tasks to complete each week. It takes months for her to achieve any fluid pattern of thought and memory recall. It's also very easy to measure every memory slip as a negative related to brain injury when it's our very nature to forget things from time to time. I must continue to remind myself of this as we work through Rosie's recovery.

I liaise with her team regarding the support I can give and adding to the regular daily conversation, memory rebuilding and domestic assistance, we slot in regular supported walks around the caravan park. There are short strolls on the cliffs interspersed with little excursions out to town. We practise walking inside, carrying trays and mugs of tea. It takes a succession of tiny steps for her to turn just 180 degrees. It's incredibly challenging for Rosie and she struggles with the coordination of more than a couple of tasks together. She continues to laugh at herself as she tries hard to marry together her cognition and mobility.

"One soup and another soup, Sir? Madame?" 'The Waitress' – Julie Walters' iconic sketch: we have watched this classic comedy so many times since your accident and laughed so much. It resonates with your current situation and you see the comedy in the things you can and can't do. I think it helps you, my love, to laugh, and to overcome the things that could so easily make you cry. It's a blessing to have this unique ability. It will support you in your healing, I know it will.

Rosie's rehab assistant's main priority is to offer her support with walking outside. As she starts to attempt walking more independently, she develops a real anxiety and fear when walking without aid. This is possibly due to the massive subconscious trauma she has deep within her brain and body from the impact of her accident. Rosie can literally freeze with fear and sometimes she just sits down on the ground unable to move, completely overtaken by distress and by frustration with herself. When we go to the supermarket, Rosie is unable to even push the trolley back from the car to the trolley park. Crossing the internal supermarket roadway is impossible. I try and insist that she does this but I support her back to the car afterwards, thinking that the more she does this, the more her confidence to do it by herself will increase.

She works through these challenges with the guidance of her psychologist and we make little gains. Still she perseveres, repeating the same routes over again. I remember a time when she sat down on the sofa in fear and just cried her eyes out, telling us she would never be able to walk outside again because of the way she felt. We had to do something to help her move on from this scary place so we introduce a stick to support her walking outside and this certainly helps her confidence. Sometimes she feels comfortable without it and sometimes she needs it constantly for reassurance.

After explaining Rosie's situation to a friend experienced in the rehabilitation of ex-servicemen, he offers advice and guidance. He suggests we make use of the swimming pool on the caravan park so a plan of regular sessions using upper body floats, balls and leg weights is drawn up. This aims to help improve her walking in a very safe environment with the main purpose being to give her confidence, build up her muscle tone and improve her brain function. I carry out these sessions twice a week or as often as Rosie is able, and we have a lot of fun. I push her as much as she pushes herself during these sessions, although her fatigue often gets the better of her, but we persist over the weeks and improvements start to be made.

It still takes so much effort for her to carry out simple exercises due to her brain injury and physical challenges and it's hard for us both to stop our frustration at times. Patience somehow has to be found in bucketloads to move forward.

As you come back to us, I sometimes see how difficult it is for you but can't imagine just how hard it must be, your frustration with your situation getting the better of you and my sadness with your situation often getting the better of me. You are trying so much to find yourself again in amongst this disarranged present, this convoluted place and time that you are in. Each day makes a difference, you get stronger and stronger. I think I can see that more than you can ...

The approach of mid-summer sees us now well-acquainted with the weekly pattern of therapist visits, assessments and swimming sessions. As time goes on, Rosie retains a little more information but still struggles to recall the events from the day before, although sometimes she astounds us with information she has retained.

Her iPhone and iPad prove invaluable as aids to Rosie and her daily selection of brain improvement games are done religiously and without fail, such is her determination to improve. I receive an immense boost of encouragement when told by someone with personal experience of brain injury to expect sudden leaps of progress from time to time as the brain makes its improvements, and we hope this will prove the case with Rosie. The key is repetition, repetition and more repetition, sometimes of the simplest of tasks until information is retained and stored.

Department of Work and Pensions – part 1

I now have to up-skill myself with the complexities of our challenging disability benefit system on Rosie's behalf, ranging from lengthy, complicated forms to fill in to uncomfortable telephone calls and degrading face-to-face interviews. We plough on through and eventually Rosie is able to receive the financial help she deserves. It is very hard for Rosie to accept this as she has always been such a hard worker and prides herself on being financially independent, working continuously while studying to help support herself through her university years. However, this must be done for the time being.

This process is a truly onerous and ongoing task and one that takes months to sort out. I struggle with the bureaucracy of it all but I am always pleasantly surprised when issues get sorted out, and when they don't, I just think we are fortunate to live in a country that has access to a welfare system and I try to remain patient even if it is through gritted teeth at times.

I inform the DVLA of her injury and am advised that she will have to embark on a process of assessments to keep her driving licence in the future. This is some way off and can't really be a reality as things currently stand, but who knows what the future may bring?

I set about creating a filing system for the different elements of correspondence for Rosie – benefits, medical reports and appointments, brain injury team information and solicitor's communications. This helps me to keep a handle on what's happening and, as I am frequently asked for information, it is easier to lay my hands on what's needed and keep my own head as straight as is possible in the process.

Chapter 31

Last Ops and the Elusive Consultant

While the new facets of our day-to-day life at home carry on, there are still three minor operations Rosie has to undergo. Her wisdom teeth need to be removed as their position had been altered due to the impact of the accident on her face; she needs corrective surgery at Moorfields Eye Hospital for double vision; and the extensive metal work in her lower right leg is ready to be removed as it seems to be restricting her ankle movement and she is in continuous pain.

We begin a succession of regular visits to Travelodges, familiar waiting rooms and food outlets, flying back and forth to St George's once again for appointments, pre-assessments and these operations.

One particularly strange appointment we have is with the Orthopaedic Outpatients at St George's. We rock up on time for our appointment and sit and wait and wait until some hours have passed. After making inquiries we are told that Rosie's notes have been mislaid, which is hard to believe as they are bulky in size and contain the amount of paper produced from a small tree.

After a further wait, we are taken into a consulting room and are told that her consultant has gone home as he was convinced this patient could not be Rosie, basing his opinion on the fact that he last saw her in her very early critical days in intensive care and very few people in her condition make it out the other side. He thought she was dead.

Staggered and quite perturbed by this information, we arrange a further appointment to see him now that other staff can vouch for the fact that she is still very much here. When we do eventually get to see this consultant, some weeks later, he confirms his side of the story exactly and can't quite believe Rosie is sitting in front of him, very much alive.

We are still unsure of what to make of this rather odd encounter but look back and laugh at its ironic aspects from time to time. We are reminded how Rosie cheated death and how amazing her comeback really is.

Rosie takes all these operations in her stride and they seem very tame compared to what she has been through. We are constantly reminded of the past when we return to places with Rosie that we visited months ago and compare the differences in her progress. It's very odd to see her back in a hospital bed.

I sit beside your bed; you wear a familiar blue and white hospital gown such as the one you were in permanently many months ago. You are so alive now, my love, so chatty and animated and mobile as you munch away on your prawn sandwich. I can start to rewrite some of those old images in my head now, I can eradicate some of that pain and anxiousness. We have moved on from that time and you are living proof of that. You are mending now, and I am too.

Chapter 32

Roots and Wings

After a brain injury, it's quite common for survivors to become overwhelmed when they are faced with a busy street full of people and, due to spatial awareness, overload of noise and constant movement in combination with physical challenges, it can be a very uncomfortable environment. When we are in London, we often challenge Rosie, although she needs little persuasion, by taking her to Oxford Street to see how she fares. Before her accident she studied, worked and socialised in this area of London for some years so it was all very familiar to her. Although she can't remember exactly where things are at this stage of her recovery, her ability to walk through the streets, stick firmly in hand, is quite amazing. We are astounded by her tolerance, in short bursts, of bustling coffee shops and restaurants, and her ability nonetheless to decipher conversation through the constant background noise. Perhaps this is because she is young and had so many years in clubs, busy student bars and work environments. Her threshold is possibly higher than most people's although her fatigue is evident when she overdoes things.

As we walk these streets, I prompt your memories as we pass each place you knew so well. The London College of Fashion in John Prince's Street, your study campus in High Holborn, the Topshop you worked in here and the clubs you used to hang out in. It's all so vague and so muddled, isn't it? It must seem so frightening and frustrating for you that you can't place these memories back in your filing system yet, in any order or sequence of time. They may return to you one day when your healing is ready. But you must concentrate on what's important to your healing just now.

Having been thrust into such an unexpected situation at this point in my lifetime, I can feel resentful at times. I lack the freedoms and choices I once had but as we progress, I adapt as best I can, based on my instincts as a mother. I struggle to let go of my nurturing at times as Rosie's awareness and reconnections improve alongside her independence from me. I need to constantly re-evaluate my role and so I start to leave her on her own at home for the odd hour or two.

One particular day she texts me to ask if she can use up some bacon from the fridge for a sandwich for lunch. As I reply, mentioning the things to watch out for – level of gas control to prevent burning, not leaving the pan on the heat after cooking, etcetera – I suddenly realise my large vat of recently-made apple jelly is sitting on the hob, complete with its tea towel cover draping over the side and very close to the other gas rings. I suddenly feel overwhelmed with concern that Rosie may not be vigilant enough to think about the potential fire risks. I have to trust myself, though, that she will, and I refrain from texting her back to alert her to this. When I arrive home, I can see that she has carefully pushed back the pan and lifted the dangling cloth away from the gas rings. These may seem the smallest of things to worry about but when someone's injured brain is working through the simplest of processes again, they can be great indicators of how a brain is repairing.

It's hard at times as Rosie is still reliant on me, more for reassurance, memory-prompting and a small amount of physical help than anything else, which is understandable given the absolutely devastating life-changing point she is at now. She needs my companionship as she is so isolated here at home, left dangling and so remote from any life that resembles her past one.

As we move through her recovery, I sometimes feel the expected levels of achievement that come with brain injury rehabilitation can feel quite stark and rigid. There clearly has to be a benchmark to work towards and even though there are changes in a person, the premorbid aspects of that person and their life before injury must really be thoroughly considered, as we are all so unique to ourselves. The standard cake-making, kitchen tasks and domestic chores are all good if someone has always had to do these in life beforehand, but if someone's life hasn't had to incorporate these things before, it's a big ask to challenge them to do this while recovering from a brain injury. It is suggested to Rosie on one occasion that she take up a musical instrument, the violin for example. She side-lines this instantly since the last musical instrument she played was the triangle, badly, in her infant school production.

Her occupational therapist constantly thinks of new experiences that may help Rosie progress. It is difficult in this rural environment, and opportunities to meet other young people in similar situations to hers are very limited.

To get her out of the home environment, Rosie is encouraged to take a 'Mindfulness' course about an hour away from our home at the Dorset Brain Injury unit in Poole, so we add this into our weekly schedule. She is reluctant at first to take part, but after some persuasion she gives it a go for the first few sessions. However, she soon arrives at the conclusion that walking slowly across a small room avoiding others is not quite what she wants as part of her recovery plan, particularly when she has conquered Oxford Street and when there is a beautiful summer's day to be had outside. Analysing the finer details of raisins for a whole hour is clearly not her way forward either; so we knock that one on the head and think of something different, something perhaps more in tune with her nature.

A Tai Chi class in a remote village hall is suggested as a possible option that could improve Rosie's balance, so we attend, and with most of the class being retired oldies it does not feel the right place for a young person, despite her injuries. Her face says it all when I wander past the hall window and glance in, catching her eye and her frustrated expression. When the session ends we chuckle at the situation she has found herself in and agree that the options in London for her physical and social recovery may be a little more abundant than in a sleepy village in West Dorset.

"Mum can I try ballet and Mum can I go horse riding and Mum can I have singing lessons? Pleeeease." I said you could try them all, but I will make it clear, and, unlike my own mother for me, I am NOT taking you if you lose interest. The

enthusiasm waned after the first few sessions, didn't it? We laugh at that now, and how reluctant I was to exhaust myself taking you all from one thing to another, under duress. In some bizarre way It feels like we have been ricocheted back to those times, doesn't it?

As Rosie slowly improves with her walking, her stability and her memory, we see how she copes with serving customers in the caravan park reception. Her sunny disposition and excellent customer service skills were always amongst her great assets. She manages simple tasks for a couple of hours at a time: pricing, stock rotation and some computer tasks. It's a challenge to her memory and fatigue gets the better of her at times but she enjoys the change of scenery, proving to herself and others that her shop skills from the past and her professionalism and customer service are still with her despite her fuzziness. With practice, we hope she will improve further.

Rosie's main goal, which she emphatically refuses to relinquish, is to get back to work and London. Her company have been working closely with her occupational therapist and she is invited to do a couple of half days over the next few months to see how she fares, and they work hard to find an appropriate starting point. This will be a test for her but a necessary one to establish a way forward.

We feel excited for her to have something to focus on, a short-term goal for her to work towards. The thought of her returning to London in her current, rather vulnerable state is a scary thought for us. Adrian and I have never been overprotective 'cottonwool' parents and always vowed to give our children roots and wings as much as we were able to. For the moment, though, Rosie's wings are a bit battered, so our approach is that she needs to spend some time repairing them here at home, in order to fly again. We hope our chrysalis will turn again into a beautiful butterfly.

I first came across this beautiful piece of writing from 'The Prophet' by Kahlil Gibran in the early 1980s. It was given to me by a friend who I shared a flat with in London. I have loved it ever since and, even though we have winged our parenting on many occasions, I always had in mind to carry this philosophy in my heart as much as I could while bringing up our family.

*And a woman who held a babe against her bosom
   said, "Speak to us of children."*
And he said:
"Your children are not your children.
*They are the sons and daughters of Life's longing
   for itself.*
They come through you but are not from you,
*And though they are with you yet they belong not
   to you.*
You may give them your love but not your thoughts,
For they have their own thoughts.
You may house their bodies but not their souls,
*For their souls dwell in the house of tomorrow,
   which you cannot visit, not even in your dreams.*
*You may strive to be like them but seek not to make
   them like you.*

For life goes not backward nor tarries with yesterday.
You are the bows from which your children as living arrows are sent forth."

From 'The Prophet' by Kahlil Gibran

Chapter 33
Growing a Thicker Skin

The autumn months of 2015 reveal increased memory retention and Rosie's personality traits poking through. As I stand by the cooker one day I feel her arms spontaneously and so naturally encircle me and the words "I love you, Mum" so genuinely flow from her heart and through her lips, sending me into floods of tears and indicating the relationship we have with each other remaking its pre-accident connections and rekindling the closeness we once had.

Today was another of those wonderful days, a heart-bursting sort of day. "I love you, Mum..." You meant that, I know you genuinely did. I know now that all the anger and the rage you show me at times cannot override this, my love, not ever. I blot those moments out and replace them with this one because this one is the true and meaningful one and those scenes are just resentment and frustration as your brain recovers. I love you too, my darling girl, I love you more than you could ever begin to know.

As Rosie gets stronger, we go out and about each week visiting the supermarket and local town shops. We have now become so accustomed to the constant looks from strangers, but other reactions are quite different. Gawping had always been the case during the early days when Rosie came out from hospital at weekends; but being here at home, where we are known by others, gives rise to a completely different set of reactions. We have had friends and acquaintances approach us directly and kindly ask Rosie how she is doing; others avoid eye contact with her and just speak to us about her, not knowing quite how to conduct themselves in her presence. Others avoid us completely by turning down another supermarket aisle or darting conveniently into the nearest shop doorway when they see us approaching. However, sometimes I feel as though I am taking the same evasive action myself, when I am feeling sensitive and not up for engaging in conversation.

It's not that she looks much different from how she looked before her accident, apart from her slightly awkward walk and slow movement; it's the unknown that is difficult for some, which I suppose leaves them scared of what might happen. Sometimes we have been in the presence of others who constantly observe us both, forming their opinions, usually without education, and waiting for 'something to happen' which confirms in their minds that "She's not right" or "Shame, isn't it?" People can be very eager to offer their views on our situation and I'm sure it's generally with good intent. Although when someone suggests Rosie may end up in sheltered housing, I find that difficult to imagine as I am not sure what that actually means at this stage myself. It's very hard to know what to say and I think I too would have struggled, before my acquaintance with brain injury, if the boot was on the other foot.

Brain injury, of any nature, conjures up all sorts of assumptions in people's minds. After all, it affects our main control centre and it's very easy to arrive at the worst-case conclusion.

So many times, when we have been met with this variety of reactions, Rosie has echoed my thoughts instantly, articulating to me the sense she gets from others, her perception and understanding bang on the money. If only they could see behind this silent disability to the intellect that lies below, they would perhaps question the way they act. I have learnt to grow a thicker skin now but often feel more hurt than she does, with Rosie usually saying, "Don't let it affect you, Mum, it's their ignorance that holds them back."

Do you remember when we were free to leave the farm after the Foot and Mouth disease confinement ban had been lifted? Can you pluck these memories from your filing cabinet just yet? It was such a relief, wasn't it, to be back out in the outside world again, free to do as we pleased. We weren't prepared for the shuns and stares when we went to the local supermarket and town. I used to jokingly say that these people must think we have Foot and Mouth disease under our fingernails. We felt a bit like lepers then and I sometimes experience that feeling of déja vu *now.*

I feel a deep sense of isolation and loneliness at times. After the first initial influx of interest in our situation, the texts and calls taper off and the gaps between visits from other people get longer. I just long to have some respite on my own, a regular cup of tea or a listening ear to make me feel human again. This isn't where I thought I would be at this stage of my life, and I can get distracted in thought about the lives of others being much less complicated than mine. It's irrational though, as we are all equally vulnerable to life's interwoven ups and downs. These brief moments of self-pity don't last for long but I acknowledge them as part of my own healing process.

Rosie feels the same, too. Her connection with friends disappears, apart from two local friends who see her from time to time. She and I so often feel we are thought of as one now, and not as the individuals we are. We tend to stick close to some dear friends who have opened their hearts, their minds and their doors, accepting us and giving Rosie the time of day. They make her feel real again and at ease so that her wonderful quick wit and natural warmth can shine through. This incredible girl is a lesson for us all. Rarely does she complain about her lot and she jokes regularly about her shortcomings and forgetfulness in such an admirable way, it makes me careful not to complain too much about a simple headache or my midlife tiredness.

Chapter 34
Golden Cap November Milestone

Pollyanna achieved first-class honours in her degree this year, despite the last horrendous few months. She has worked so hard and earned every bit of her top grade and we are so proud of her achievements. Her graduation day arrives and we all prepare for a Winchester Cathedral ceremony and a celebratory London meal. It's such a thrill to see her receive her award and afterwards we head up to London to have our family meal in Covent Garden.

It's a very long day for Rosie but she keeps up in true Rosie style, despite the sore feet and fatigue. It's always wonderful to have a family celebration and we treasure them more than ever now. As we leave the restaurant and go on to the street a raised voice comes through the darkness towards us: "Are you Rosie? You were in the Wolfson with my Grandad!"

We all turn around in amazement. What a hoot to be recognised completely out of context, well after she has left hospital and in the dark as well!

November 2015 arrives and we say goodbye to all the caravan park holidaymakers for another season. Things quieten down a little and our thoughts turn to how our lives have changed from this time a year ago. Rosie is very keen to mark the day of her accident in a positive way so we suggest a walk up to the highest point in Dorset, Golden Cap, finishing with a fish and chip lunch at the seafront pub below it, always giving her what we think to be a greater challenge than she can master and always keen for her to prove us wrong. She is adamant that, although she feels emotional, we are not going to sit around and feel sorry for ourselves, crying into our soup.

On this November 11th day after our very poignant two-minute silence, we prepare for the day ahead. Today has its own special meaning of remembrance for us as we are truly thankful for life on so many levels.

As I pull on my shabby woollen walking socks, I remind myself of the pact I made this time last year to keep the same polish on my toenails that I painted on that evening before Rosie's accident. Superstitious perhaps, but I wanted to see just how much progress she would have made by the time it naturally disappeared. I glance at the last tiny speck that remains and inwardly express my gratitude for what we have been granted over this last year with Rosie's recovery.

We head off in Myrtle, our camper van, the weather grey and murky very like last year but the circumstances so incredibly different. Champagne, wellies and Monty at the ready, we start our ascent, the hard grind to the summit. Rosie is still walking tentatively with a stick, so we amble along slowly with Adrian supporting her at challenging points along the way. We take in the beautiful coastal scenery that surrounds us and reflect on the differences between today and the same day a whole year ago.

If we could have had a peep into the future twelve months ago from her intensive care bedside in St George's and that lowest point when that doctor said to me "But she is still breathing" to today, we would have cried with disbelief; and we look at her now, well and truly breathing, marching as fast as her legs will permit, wittily chatting away and laughing as we go.

We reach the majestic top of the Cap, a little wet and buffeted by the conditions but in no way deterred from our mission, and we crack open the fizz and raise our glasses. Rosie snaps away as she would always have done, making lasting memories of this significant day and time of her life, pictures of the progress she has made on her incredible journey.

While we celebrate, a young girl and an older women happen to pass as they walk the costal path and ask us what the occasion is: "We are celebrating Rosie's life," I reply and we exchange some words of mutual thankfulness for life itself, the young girl's for the chance she still has to walk with her much-loved elderly grandmother and ours to be exactly where we are today with our incredible daughter.

We leave the top and descend towards our lunch, with Monty leading the way and Rosie slipping and sliding a little through the muddy gateways, linked solidly to Adrian one side and to her stick the other – never giving in to the constant pain in her ankle and continuously pushing through the challenges her brain injury poses.

I happen to glance down to her feet as we near the end of our walk and suddenly realise the wellingtons Rosie is wearing are twenty-plus years old, cheap agricultural store boots costing the princely sum of around £4.99. We laugh at this – growing up on a farm had its uses; you just had to wear what was available. Rosie embraces her memorable rural roots and with stoic gusto completes today's challenge.

Now we have marked this milestone in such a notable way, acknowledged it and somehow drawn an imaginary line under it for the time being, we can move forward from this point towards the future.

A year ago today was a very different day, my love, when we were all thrust into a different world, an hour to hour, day to day existence of angst. I used to pinch myself then to confirm that our living hell was a reality and I am doing just that today, too, but in such a different way as I watch you climb the Cap the way you are. You are now what our hope gave us then. You have climbed another sort of hill this year from those moments where death was so nearly your only option to this place now which represents nature's powerful best, the blending life energy of sea and land. Let's harness this power and carry it forward to next year. I think you have so much more life to live...

Chapter 35
First Steps to Independence

Rosie is asked to meet an old friend in Exeter for lunch so I suggest she catch the train on her own from Axminster, a straightforward, half-hour journey that she had done on many occasions, and her friend would meet her at the other end. With her anxiety for walking on pavements at its highest, she feels doubtful that she could complete this task despite the continuous use of her stick. Her memory is still very sketchy, and she struggles to visualise the once familiar places in the city and has serious doubts about her ability to ever achieve this. Her injury has left her more cautious, physically slower and less mobile, which in turn can make her a bit vulnerable on her own in busy situations. After much deliberation, she decides to embrace the challenge and we organise the day ahead. Rosie knows deep down this has to be attempted for her to start the next phase towards independence and I wholeheartedly agree. We verbally repeat the route until she is confident about the procedure and the stop to get off at and I see her onto the train. My feeling of apprehension is intense to say the least as I envisage all manner of things going wrong – Rosie ending up in Penzance being one of them.

As I tearfully leave the station, I receive a text message from her confirming with me again the stop to get off and letting me know that she is seated next to a nice lady and they are having a chat. We are both reassured.

I have to remind myself of my parenting now. You were free to roam the farm, playing in the straw bales, sliding down the bank in the bluebell wood on old bits of corrugated iron sheets; Pollyanna still bears the scar where the sharp edge gouged her leg. And that awful slurry pit; I showed you on our daily walks the best way to walk safely past it. That day when you and Edd, as tots, escaped from the house down to the tractor shed, I immediately panicked thinking you would have fallen or thrown yourselves in like it was a swimming pool; but children don't generally put themselves in danger when they are aware of those dangers. I found you both happily engrossed in the tractors. You know from that tender age we encouraged you to understand what danger was but also allowed you to 'feel your fear' so that you could make decisions for yourselves, to become independent in your thinking. This has stood you in good stead for today, my love; you have pushed yourself through your fear and achieved what you set out to do and I admire you for that.

After an enjoyable few hours in town with her old friend and having completed the journeys without a hitch, Rosie is back home and chatting about her day as much as she can remember, her first taste of independence boosting her confidence no end. After this, Rosie takes the bus a few times to Bridport to meet her rehab assistant and to practise orientation, walking with confidence and road crossing. This is still such a challenge for her, but she completes these tasks and starts to relearn some old skills and lay down some new.

Her Speech and Language therapist is happy with her current progress and now leaves Rosie to build on her existing memory and speech which improves slowly week by week. Rosie continues religiously with her daily brain activities on her iPad, increasing her vocabulary and word-finding skills. She continually asks us to help her fill in the gaps of her missing months, retaining more as time goes on. Her phone is permanently in use as her memory aid and we regularly assist by adding little prompts for her to kickstart her cognitive wheels which in turn help her memory flow and her recall to improve.

Rosie can often get confused when her fatigue or cognitive functioning takes an overload but she resists the advice to rest sometimes. Her old memories are sometimes easier to recall than her new ones, but we hope this will improve as time heals her.

Her first work experience morning at her old company is planned for early December so we head up to London. It's good for her to spend time with her old colleagues and she naturally slots into the office banter again, recognising everyone she worked with. However, Rosie still can't recall her old work tasks and, even though a lot of her computer skills are still intact, her memory and slow processing speed hamper the many administrative skills she once had. It's not easy being so far away in Dorset for her to ease back into her type of work here and, as her brain still has so much healing to do, she is unable to keep testing herself and her abilities. Her HR team constantly look for other opportunities both within her company and externally and suggest it might be beneficial for her to come up to London for a two-week stint in the new year. An offer of some work experience at the JoJo Maman Bébé headquarters in Battersea is suggested as a start; and this gives Rosie a goal for next year to look towards.

Chapter 36

2016 – Show Us What You've Got!

As Christmas approaches this year, I reflect upon our last as much as my memory allows. This year will signify again the progress Rosie has made in her recovery and will be a chance for us all to touch base with our own feelings and make progress with rebuilding our family unit.

It's been hard for all of us to make some adjustments but harder still for Rosie. As she repairs, she grows through the different stages of her rebirth and is heading towards her mid-twenties again. She never ceases to amaze us all with her recovery and is often a much calmer and more philosophical version of her old self although she too, like her siblings when they all get together, tends to do as most offspring do when they come back to the family nest – revert to the behaviour they had as kids. It needs to happen to re-establish these relationships that perhaps in time will have a more meaningful significance. It's great to have everyone together and our home is filled, just as it always has been – with the obvious exception of last year – with laughter, fun, games and merriment. The routines are reinstated and traditions upheld, with Rosie one hundred percent cashing in on the fact that she missed out last year.

We spend New Year celebrating and wonder how far she will have come by this time next year. There is no doubt that this next year will be far less eventful than the last and we hope it will open its doors to Rosie's independence and her new life.

Rosie's New Year resolution is to ditch the stick. She has started to have periods of keeping it in her handbag when out and about and giving herself walking challenges. Her confidence is helped by weekly yoga sessions and some treadmill hits. Now that she is conquering her anxiety and progressing well, I offer her a proposition. Rosie has been keen for some time to don her trainers and running gear to see what she can do. We work out a short route around the flattest bit of the caravan park and start.

This is far more of a challenge than we thought but, as she builds up her fitness, she starts to make small gains. Her brain and body evidently work very much harder than before. Understandably, Rosie gets frustrated about her slow pace, since before her accident she would have been able to crack out an eight-mile run at an average pace of eight and a half minutes a mile and barely looked as though she had broken sweat. Her fatigue now is immense just for the short jog she has attempted. She still has infinite determination, though, and may still be able to run the Bath half marathon with her father for which they were both training before her accident. She hopes to be able to run for charity in the future – I can't wait to be cheering her on.

It's increasingly discouraging for Rosie, particularly when she wants to keep so positive, to come to terms with life as it is at the moment. Her sadness at her current situation often increases her frustration but also fuels her desire to return to the life she once had. As a mother, it's hard to see your children struggle when their lives are at rock bottom and there is really nothing you can do.

Our family as a whole needs space to rebuild and this is increasingly hard for us all to do at such a distance, but we keep the connections going and treasure the times we have together as a family. You 'sticky tape', 'parcel tape' and 'gaffer tape' through the family rehabilitation bonding process after such a devastating time in the hope that the foundations of family stay intact. It's a rocky road at times, the sort that tears families apart. Sometimes you can't help wondering if your family will ever be truly happy again; but I have learnt to just stand back and let time heal the difficulties, and mostly this seems to work. We all have our individual acceptance to work through and I hope that we may eventually all appreciate just how much we have achieved to keep our family together as time moves on.

I cry for you all now, my children; I want to scoop you all up in my arms and hold you close to me. This is not how I imagined life to be for us all. These separate existences, the strain I see on your faces as you witness the effects of this challenging and unwelcome time. We must keep communicating and moving with hope towards a better future, when we can see more on our horizons than the devastating effects that life-changing accidents can have. I believe we are still strong, I have never really doubted that. I love you all so deeply and I am here for you too. I hope you have never doubted that either.

E... is for embrace
April 2016 – July 2019

Chapter 37

London: the Start

Therapist visits continue into January 2016 and, as Rosie is still very determined to head back to 'the Smoke', we start to plan for the pre-arranged two-week work experience in Battersea. We find a comfortable flat to rent in Southfields and plan our trip. Rosie will be working for a few hours each morning and assisting in different departments, giving her a taster of each and a chance to be part of an office again.

We settle in and plan bus times, shopping time and down time. It's great to see Rosie back in her old mode again and, although still gaining her strength, her zest for city life is never too far away and nor is her determination to unearth those routines that she left off so abruptly in November 2014. Yes, she needs me as her constant support just now and our relationship inevitably remains very close, but she proves that the more she can do on her own, the more her sense of independence will return. By the end of the two weeks we execute our morning routines like clockwork, Rosie often ahead of schedule as her desire to get back to routine is top priority.

I accompany her to and from work each day and we gradually factor in some mornings when she catches the first bus back after work from Battersea and I follow on the next one, setting herself the stop to meet me at and using her City Mapper app to aid her. We build on this over the two weeks and she copes incredibly well. We make friends with the waitress in the Power Station café which we have now designated our regular morning coffee stop before Rosie starts work, and I familiarise myself with the area.

I spend my mornings walking in and around Battersea Park, watching the array of humans and wildlife that are in abundance here. I frequently see dog walkers from the Dogs' Refuge and wonder if they would like a spare set of hands for a few hours. It's late February so the winter still has its firm grip, but the weather is kind to me, and the coffee shops welcoming, offering interludes of warmth and solace.

During a period of down time, Rosie and I decide to have a hairdresser treat one afternoon; and on the bus on our way back from the Southside shopping centre, we encounter a rather uncomfortable experience.

As we sit close to the back of the busy bus near a group of exuberant youngsters, I feel a sharp tug at my hair. After the second or third tug, I turn to the group and firmly suggest they stop, only to be met with a reactive kick on the back of my leg. I instantly feel unnerved by this situation, vulnerable myself and responsible for Rosie. My emotions get the better of me and my tears start to roll down. Rosie, aware of this, starts to talk to the boys but they continue their 'mouthing off' to her so she, along with the kind young girl who I am sitting next to, suggests we get off at the next stop, thus defusing any further antagonism.

I sit for a moment or two on the bus stop bench to compose myself, Rosie and this lovely girl calming me down and all of us agreeing how despicable the lads' behaviour had been. Rosie's street-wise traits and the protective side of her nature towards her rather pathetic, blubbering, middle-aged mother revealed themselves in characteristic fashion.

This moment was in some way a turning point for me as she comforted me through the dark streets back to our flat. Rosie not only proved, as she has done on a number of occasions before, that she looks out for my wellbeing as well as her own, just as she had always done, but also that she is still able to cope with a situation like this one without being fazed.

I feel reassured that, as time goes on and her healing improves, she will be back to this city life she did not choose to leave; maybe with a different direction from the one she had before, but it definitely feels right for her to be given the chance again and I am not going to stand in her way, however hard it will be for me to let her go again. But I must.

After receiving a lovely send-off from Rosie's newly-acquainted office colleagues who have clearly been affected by her warmth and personality, we head back to Dorset to plan her next steps.

As the year starts to unfold, we have to embark upon the legal process to build the case for Rosie against the insurance company of the car driver. Her legal team inform us that she will have to have many intense assessments over the next few years with a range of medico-legal professionals to examine the full extent of her injuries and determine how they will impact her future. We are now at the start of one of the longest and hardest stretches of all our lives. The impact on us all is something we are so unprepared for.

As we wade through the many appointments, I start to think frequently about the people who assisted Rosie on the day of her accident. She has often said she would like to meet them to thank them in person, so we arrange for her to meet the police and some of the staff at St George's, giving them a chance to fill us all in on some of the details of the events of that morning and for them to see just how much progress Rosie has made.

I have often wondered about the man who went to her aid on that day and what he saw. It really starts to niggle away at me, and I start my quest to contact him. I eventually manage to find an address and compose a letter to him, conveying our thanks and suggesting, if he felt up for it, that we arrange for him to meet Rosie.

One evening, shortly after my letter was posted, the phone rang. As it rang, both Adrian and I had a strong feeling that this gentleman was at the other end of the phone. Indeed he was; and, after briefly chatting, we arranged to meet him over a coffee.

It was a very emotional couple of hours for us all. He filled us in on his recollections of that morning and what he did for Rosie, lying down beside her and talking to her. He had recently watched a programme that touched on the importance of talking to someone to keep them alive at the scene of an accident, unaware then that he was about to put that information well and truly into practice. We are sure it absolutely saved her from shutting down and dying.

He recounted that he continued with his day and caught the train to his work immediately after caring for Rosie and sat in his shocked state, his shirt now covered in Rosie's blood. He jokingly said that Rosie owed him a new shirt as it was a write-off! For the years that followed, as he travelled daily past the accident scene, he would regularly think about her. I feel that perhaps he can draw a line under that day now, knowing that what he did was an exceptional act of kindness; and meeting Rosie can only have helped this.

Springtime approaches and as the caravan park opens its doors for another season, we celebrate a family Easter centred around our big event this year: Edd and Dani's wedding. Preparations are gathering momentum, suitable venues being selected, bridesmaids' dress designs circulated, decorations discussed, and invitations made. The hen and stag 'dos' are planned to take place a few weeks prior to the wedding. The list for Edd and Dani of things they need to accomplish before their big day is endless.

Rosie's physical challenges continue to improve, and she will now be able to take her place walking proudly behind Dani. What a day to look forward to in so many ways for us all.

As Rosie improves, she realises that life may not be quite the same as it was; but equally, it is a whole lot better than it could have been. We tick along most days, but with her therapies tailing off now, Rosie's boredom and sense of isolation grow. Her frustration with being stuck in Dorset and not getting back to London life increases and her desire to return to London gets more and more desperate. We are unsure how this will ever happen. However, Rosie has proved us wrong on so many levels before when we may have doubted her; so we go along with her wishes as her wings pick up their speed and we support her in her wish to return.

I wish I knew how to change your life for you, but I don't, my love, I search myself for suggestions, and I know they are not what you want. You want your life back, but you need to heal too. These next years for you will be tough and I am not sure how we will cope, but we will. Let's go and search for the opportunities that will prepare you for each step towards the life you desire.

Being at home with her parents is starting to grate and rightly so, but she has needed this for her recovery and will still need this as part of her return plan. Things have to be built on, and slowly, but Rosie is impatient, so we look at possibilities to get her back over the coming months. Her determination is phenomenal and our hunt for suitable rooms starts alongside her rehabilitation transfer from the Dorset Brain Injury Service to the St John's Therapy Centre in Wandsworth, London which is linked to St George's Hospital.

It's such a contrast living in Dorset for someone who needs to return to test her independence as Rosie does. With few transport links and her siblings and some old friends away in London, she feels very isolated and cut off from reality at times. After a bit of searching, a temporary house share is found through a flatshare website in a convenient street close to Southfields village centre. We move her back at the end of May to start the next steps towards achieving her independence.

We felt sick leaving you today, my love. I don't think you realise just how fragile you still are. You are gutsy, I know that, but your healing still needs to be tended gently; like a garden full of emerging spring flowers, you need the right conditions to blossom and bloom. Please allow this and be compassionate towards yourself as you tread the path to your new life and acceptance.

Rosie gently settles back into life in London, supported by her brain injury team, and progresses through relearning and regaining some of her independence. Her rehab assistant sets her challenges on London Transport. She learns to do the cooking, washing and cleaning for herself again with the support of her occupational therapist and rehab assistant. Adrian and I are at the end of the phone when she needs reassurance and support, which she often does when her memory lets her down. She courageously and vehemently will not be beaten, rarely giving in to challenges and continually pushing herself.

As the summer months arrive, we have our family wedding, a truly wonderful day with Rosie walking with the other bridesmaids behind Dani up the church aisle and towards the most beautiful of unions. During the reception speeches, Rosie is presented with a single stem of white gladiolus, the flower that represents strength of character; I don't think anyone can argue with that.

July also sees the last of our children's graduation ceremonies and it is another proud family moment as we see Will graduate at the Royal Festival Hall. Rosie too had her graduation ceremony at this great hall, although her memory of this day in 2014 is still quite hard for her to fully recall. It's another lovely day, marked in our traditional way by a family celebratory meal.

Rosie's strength of character is in evidence after she pays a visit to Edd and Dani's house. Rosie catches the train from Bishops Stortford to Liverpool Street, incorporating two different tube journeys on her route back to Southfields and towing a heavy suitcase all on her own. She signs up for the local gym and has a personal trainer for support, making progress with her walking and confidence.

We frequently visit her to take her to various appointments associated with her court case and although on each occasion we see improvements, we wonder how long she can sustain the pace, as she still tires very easily and her memory is still a constant battle for her. Rosie's workplace has now exhausted all opportunities for her so sadly she will have to explore other options and her funds won't sustain her forever.

After a few months, the NHS brain injury team feel they have done all they can for her in London so we are stuck as to how to move her forward without having the right funding and appropriate support.

There is a bit of me that feels you are not quite ready for this, my love; it is a great test for you. I know London is in your heart; I have never questioned that. Home is always here if you need it again, a backstop, a place of sanctuary to tend those wings again if you need to. I will leave this up to you, darling girl.

Chapter 38

The Respite Return

And so, in late autumn of 2016, Rosie makes the decision to return to Dorset for some respite. We all agree that her six month stay in London was the test she needed to prove that it's what she wants for her future. Once her case is finalised, she will be able to get the right finetuning support she needs to progress. Her long-term goal is still firmly set.

We decide to mark this year's November 11th anniversary by taking a short break to Nice. This will be Rosie's first flight since her accident and a test for the scanners to see if they pick up the large amount of metalwork in her face; but she passes through without a hitch. We have a great few days, taking the slow and rickety costal bus from Nice to Monte Carlo for an anniversary lunch on the actual day.

As Rosie adjusts to being back in Dorset and we start 2017, we continue much as we did before she left for her short stint in London, with daily exercise routines; and I introduce some short runs around the local playing fields. This can make Rosie very frustrated as she can't make the improvements she would like, and I don't have the specific knowledge as to how to help her progress. She regularly pushes herself despite being at a very low ebb now; her frustrations and the long wait for any funding make life feel quite desperate for her.

We all feel a deep sense of being trapped by the legal timeline of her case and have no idea when or if she will be able to have access to funds to move her forward. We have no choice but to stick with it; and I keep her company and try my best to keep her spirits buoyant, but her desire to return to London never seems to wane.

I know you are so frustrated; you watch your life pass by you daily with no plans in place for your future. These years that should be so productive for you are spent in a vacuum; the pause button seems to have been pressed and stuck solid. I can't imagine how this must feel when you are so ready to take the next step. You keep improving but you don't see this. I know the constant berating you give yourself is deep frustration and anger. I hate it so much when you call yourself a brain-injured retard and you think I think that too; but I don't and never could. We must hold on to hope that your life will get better, my love. Life will change because that's what life does, and your independence will return; but we must make life as bearable as possible for the here and now.

I make enquiries about her driving and we start the assessment process in Exeter. She proves that she can still drive a car but is incredibly cautious and her brain struggles to process the speeds of other cars coming towards her on faster roads. She feels more confident driving in more built-up areas where the traffic is generally slower. Sadly, the right support for her isn't available here so this has to be put on the back burner for the moment. I hope that when she gets back to London permanently, she can access the proper support she needs to regain her licence. Her brain needs to improve much further for her to be able to conquer this life skill that she has lost.

We continue with the arduous rounds of appointments relating to her court case, travelling the length and breadth of the country; and we are introduced to some incredibly knowledgeable people at the top of their games in their chosen fields. From the vast number of disciplines related to neurology, to plastic surgeons, orthopaedic and vestibular specialists and many more, we upskill ourselves on many aspects of the legal system as well as of brain injury.

One particular expert really stood out for us and the advice he gave us really helped to turn Rosie's recovery around in a big way. This wonderful and experienced man was a consultant in balance and ear conditions at a clinic in Great Portland Street. He suggested that due to her accident, Rosie has had a disruption to the signal system within her ear that is responsible for balance, and that her brain compensates for this by overusing her visual sense to walk. We have often observed her looking down and concentrating hard when she walks, so this made real sense. He suggested that when a person improves on their core strength, posture and fitness, particularly with suitable exercises specifically to aid brain injury recovery, they naturally start to walk again using their whole body subconsciously. In Rosie's case, this can free up the working part of her brain to concentrate on other things, for example looking where she is going and at what she is doing.

I decide to encourage Rosie to visit an old friend who has experience as a personal trainer and knowledge about rehabilitation of brain conditions and physical difficulties. After overcoming some reluctance, Rosie embarks on regular twice-weekly sessions; and fortunately, because she is fit and young, the effects are almost instant. She works incredibly hard to improve and can now do so many more things with more fluidity and ease. The combined physical and cognitive tasks she completes regularly have had a remarkable effect on her brain injury recovery. Her memory starts to make small consistent improvements and she becomes much sharper in her recall. Her body starts to loosen up and becomes much more fluid in movement as her confidence in herself and her own ability grows. The glances from others start to lessen and this really benchmarks the progress she has made. It really has been one of those leaps in her recovery.

Our family life still functions as best it can, despite it often feeling as though we have two contrasting dimensions in time and place. We feel so desperate for Rosie to feel more equal again to her siblings as their own lives move on. We can't change what's happened but hope the gap will lessen once she is able to find herself again in her own life. Her siblings, too, feel so helpless with the current situation.

One thing that has been lovely to witness is how people who have only met Rosie since her accident accept her difficulties. This helps to bridge the gaps in a subtle way, there being no comparisons to anything other than how Rosie is now. And even though we are fortunate to still have so much of Rosie as she was before her accident, it does help us all to see this and to question our own views and feelings as we all move towards acceptance.

We regularly get the family together when we can, to help the healing process for all of us. This year, 2017, Adrian and I celebrate our milestone 30th wedding anniversary with a quiet family holiday in Marrakech. It's the tonic we all need, as my grandma would have said; and a day spent at a water park is the perfect situation, in that any sibling differences are barely noticeable. Rosie is tested with the flumes and slides; the adrenaline junkie is back throwing herself into the day with her trademark vitality and spirit, although her fatigue somewhat robs her of these at the end of each day.

Chapter 39
The Legal Slog Continues…

We carry on through weeks and months that have now turned into years of waiting as stoically as we can for the legal judgement. This has been one of the most difficult periods for us to endure. Our whole family has been on trial. When the car hit Rosie on that day, the ricocheting effects of it hit us all in one way or another. We have all been interviewed, recorded, cross-examined and had reports written about us, an intrusion that has been so unwanted. Adrian and I have often felt that our parenting and the way our family life functions have been analysed and scrutinised. I can see so clearly how this whole process can turn a brain injury survivor against their family and the family against the survivor. It is the pressure and strain that can snap the bonds if you let it. We have all made it to this point because it has been so crucial to us all to keep the family together, but it takes courage, hard work and a lot of patience.

The insurance company are reluctant to engage positively with Rosie's legal team at this stage. She is just another number on a spreadsheet that they hope will disappear without causing a big dent to their finances. They claim that she is fully able to work and live independently, thus continuing with her life as it was before her accident. Her legal team are fighting to get liability established so that Rosie can start to get some interim payments to help her return to London with the right support that she needs. The insurance company are hoping that we will accept a paltry settlement on her behalf which would be sufficient for her life and needs going forward. It isn't. We have no idea what her future needs will be. Without full-time work and a pension, her life could be very challenging indeed. She needs a positive outcome to her claim in order to secure a stable future.

We are ground down now, at the ends of our tethers; bone-tired and emotionally exhausted. We are just not used to living in such close proximity to each other for such a long stretch of time and we all selfishly crave our own space and freedoms again.

I struggle daily, watching Rosie as her young life ticks away before my eyes. She has missed four and a half years of 'living' in her twenties, a very critical part of a young person's life. Adrian and I have missed this time, too, but we are in our fifties, so it is not as bad for us. Rosie is desperate to start her life again properly, in the knowledge that she does not have to return to Dorset and with the long-term funds to make a life for herself. She craves finding her sense of purpose again, being able to fill the voids that she has with some meaningful work, leisure time and socialising, and picking up some of the threads from her life before her accident to make her feel herself again. Although Rosie has a strong affection for Dorset, she finds it hard to feel enthusiastic about life here, since it is not her choice. She has incredible resilience to keep going with her daily routines of exercise, her brain games and walking Monty. Many people in her dire situation would not have the impetus to even get out of bed in the morning.

Monty has been Rosie's most constant companion during these past years. The best therapy can come from the animals we love. At times, when Rosie feels very low, knowing that she must get out and walk him each day has kept her mental health from declining. Every day she has memory challenges, and these will be with her for life; but she religiously makes detailed notes on her phone to support herself for each day. This is now key to her functioning, and she would be lost without it. Organisation has always been one of her strong points and, thankfully, this strength remains with her. She now spends a lot of her time researching as much as she can about brain injury through the Headway website, and this helps her make progress in working towards acceptance. Understanding that others experience similar problems does offer some degree of comfort to her, I think. Identifying with others can benefit her enormously; and reading the uplifting words of her long-time inspirational heroes, such as Katie Piper, have made her feel less alone at this desperately lonely point of her life.

One thing I have found that has helped me immensely, as I have had anxiety and a nervous tic for many years, has been regular meditation. I have practised yoga for some years now and had often thought deeper meditation rather self-indulgent. That is until now. About four years ago I discovered a really practical, no-frilly-nonsense app called Headspace and can honestly say it has saved my mental health. Each morning after I wake, I sit quietly for fifteen minutes, choosing a course from the app library that I feel could help an area of emotion, and I am guided through the practice with constant, comforting support. After some years of practice, I have come to really understand the benefits and would recommend this as a simple and effective way to support yourself whether going through a difficult period in life or just to keep mentally well. It's an alternative that can work given regular time and discipline and can definitely be a way to address your mental state of mind before taking the more common medical alternatives.

I have often found the GPs eager to dish out medication, particularly when you relay to them the details of what you are having to cope with. It can be difficult to refuse when you are really at rock bottom. This approach does, however, work for many people, so I could never discount the use of this type of conventional medication; especially as I used it myself many years ago after a bout of post-natal depression, when it helped get me through a difficult patch in my life.

I have found, after being faced with challenging times such as these, that my outlook on life can sometimes get distorted. It feels on occasions as though I reach a point when I fear that every difficult thing that happens, however small, could have disastrous consequences. It's a fear that comes attached to the trauma, I think. What I feel helps is to work towards having a more balanced view of life. Good and bad things happen, but it's how we approach each event that can keep things in perspective.

One massive thing I have learnt through this is that I am not responsible for my children's happiness now that they are adults. I have always felt that I should make every wrong right for them, should be able to ease any pain that they have; and consequently, I have so often worried myself sick. Now that they are adults, I have chosen to let go of that child-nurturing a bit and recognise, as this has taught me, that some things are totally out of my power to control and change. We all have to be responsible for our own happiness in life and the only thing we can really do is remain as kind to ourselves and to others as much as we possibly can.

I also try to keep my physical exercise going as much as possible. I ran short distances on a regular basis before Rosie's accident to keep old age and senility at bay. During these last years I have found myself in many contrasting places and situations and have had to adapt accordingly, trying things I can occupy myself with in the time I have available: a brisk walk, a short run or just a quiet coffee shop with the daily newspaper or my book. When I take Rosie to her personal trainer, I have an hour to kill. I use this time to do a short run, really a gentle jog, along the Seaton esplanade. This long length of flat pavement offers a beautiful seascape and a chance to switch off as I run, accompanied by some favourite music.

When I'm running I often observe a particular man, a sad man whose face and posture exude deep pain. It bothers me, his pain, and I wonder what his story is. He walks purposefully every day and pauses when he comes to the end of the esplanade, looking out to sea in the deepest of thought. I can see and feel his pain as I run with my own; I know that feeling, not as he sees it, though, but in a different way. He had a new coat for Christmas; I hope this keeps him warm as he walks with his pain. He shuts everyone out, I think; I tried to smile at him once. I am only here temporarily so won't see him walk for much longer. I feel for this man.

Many of these places that I would not normally spend time in have become the norm now. I have had to shape my life according to the time and place of Rosie's recovery and I have realised I am much better at adjusting to change than I ever thought possible. I guess it has been a case of having to, and you never know the strengths you have until you need to dig this deep.

Department of Work and Pensions – part 2

As Rosie's recovery continues, and the benefit system changes to Universal Credit, she is asked to attend appointments to assess if she is still entitled to claim. There is no doubt that her improvements since her first assessment have altered the findings from her initial claim. However, we are quite shocked to find her PIP (Personal Independence Payment, the old Disability Living Allowance) is to be stopped. This is how it happens: we attend an assessment meeting in Axminster in an empty building on a cold January day. The half-interested assessor is clearly filled with cold and gives us the impression that this is the last thing she would rather be doing. She fires away her basic questions, barely making eye contact with Rosie during the assessment. Rosie is asked to carry out the elemental physical exercises and the standard, remembering three things and a simple maths subtraction.

The letter she subsequently receives states a number of reasons for the discontinuation of her benefit, and here are a few:

"You did not report any loss of consciousness."
"You did not look tired."
"You looked well presented."
"You can walk 200 metres."

After a further few months she attends an assessment for her Employment Support Allowance. As she is leaving the room at the end of an appointment similar to the one for her PIP assessment, the advisor calls her back and says, "Excuse me, did you say it was brain injury?" Shortly after this assessment she receives a call to say this benefit will stop as from the day of this call, and these are some of the reasons:

> *"You can deal with people you don't know."*
> *"You can stay in one place for more than an hour without having to move."*
> *"You behave in a way that would be acceptable at work" (this one still makes me feel exasperated).*

As the benefit system has changed, Rosie is advised to appeal if she does not agree with the decision, or reapply for Universal Credit.

How can an assessor arrive at these conclusions when they have only met someone for twenty minutes? Every indication points to the fact that this system has no provision to assess people who have a silent disability. It is not fit for purpose. People with silent disabilities are completely stuck in a system that does not acknowledge and cannot assess them correctly. The difficulties fluctuate daily for someone living with a brain injury; each day is different, which I acknowledge can make it difficult to assess.

When we do eventually get the appointment to attend her appeal against the loss of her PIP (over eighteen months from when it was taken away), it was humiliating and scary, to say the least. We sat for over an hour and a half in a courtroom being cross-examined by a judge, a disability professional and a medical expert. Adrian and I felt as though we were on trial as parents, and it was utterly degrading for Rosie. It was deemed that if Rosie could understand a single complex sentence, if she could use Google maps to orientate her outside and if she could wash and dress herself, then she could do without this benefit. Needless to say, Rosie's benefit was not reinstated.

I can't imagine how difficult it is for people to survive financially when things take this long to come to court and without the support of family or friends. The benefits she has received to date have paid for her personal trainer, which has helped her dramatically, as well as for her private psychology. And yes, Rosie has good support from her family and may potentially be able to access some form of work when she has funds to pay for support; but so many people don't have this. Change in this archaic, rigid, 'one size fits all' system has somehow got to take place to make this a fairer system for all.

As we enter 2018, the initial part of Rosie's court case starts to come together; all the evidence is in and the legal teams now prepare for the court date early next year to establish primary liability.

We still have such a long wait ahead of us and the frustrations we all have become very difficult to deal with. We all want our lives to move on: for Rosie to be able to start her life again and for Adrian and me to rebuild our lives together. Occasionally, each of us can let the intensity of the situation get the better of us.

There, I have done it! My glass of red wine smashes against the white wall in front of me. The feathery, blood-red sprays trickle down into every uneven nook and cranny of the wall. The wall now resembles the aftermath of a firework, a peacock fan of red and white; and I am calm, the release is immense. I am sorry, but I had to do it, to stop the tension, to change the vibe. I cleaned up my mess, that evening and into the next day. I painted over the stains and the cracks; not a vestige left behind, no sign that I had lost my composure for that brief moment. Papering over the cracks: is this something we all do from time to time? Covering up what's underneath our surface, to keep in what should occasionally be let out? We are good at that, us humans, holding it all in. It feels good to sometimes let things out.

I wasn't proud of this moment. It is not in my nature generally to act like this, but we can't judge. We are all susceptible to the fragilities of our humanness when the challenges of life get the better of us. Things just happen. There had been a few times when I wondered how it would feel to throw my glass of wine at the wall; would it release these years of pain in some way? It wasn't an angry throw; quite the opposite, really, as I was calm. It was a throw of release and relief. A lot of the pain in me went with that glass of wine as it hit the wall on that day and I felt freed up in so many ways. Afterwards, though; I hadn't quite calculated the effort I would have to produce in the clear-up stage.

After that evening of explosions, wine-related and others, it felt as though a finale had arrived to the many tense moments we have had. We have found a calmer approach, a point of consciously stopping when the heat is turned up, punctuating by inserting a pause into our periodical outbursts of the past. We have grown throughout these years, the three of us together.

As we move through this year, our family life reaches another wonderful phase. We have the delightful privilege of welcoming beautiful Willow Annie into our family. The next generation of little people and the next phase for Adrian and me as we embrace grandparenthood. There is nothing to compare with what the introduction of this new little life has brought to us all as a family. She has helped to repair our bonds more than we could ever have thought possible. I watch Willow sometimes as she grows, as her brain wakes up to the world around her, and I see the similarities between the recovery of a brain after injury and the natural development of a tiny new forming brain. Our brains are phenomenal in the power they have to both grow and to heal and the nurture we give them in both instances is crucial to their potential. We are such incredible beings from birth to death and everything in between.

The summer months are here again, and Rosie has made such good physical progress, she decides to give paddle-boarding a try in the bay at Lyme Regis. This is a very challenging activity for even the more able; but for someone recovering from a brain injury, it requires an immense amount of perseverance, particularly when it comes to balance. Rosie manages to improve during her sessions and, when the sea is calmer, she manages to stand on her board for a bit, punting away.

I am sitting cross-legged on the North Wall that overlooks Lyme Bay, watching you on your paddleboard, and I'm snapping away, taking videos for you to see what you have achieved. You used to throw yourself off this North Wall countless times into the sea after school and in the holidays during your younger years. The famous Cobb wall reaches out its majestic arm to protect its smaller counterpart and the generations upon generations of youngsters that have used this wall in that way. I still have to pinch myself in situations like this, when I remind myself just how far you have come in this chapter of your life's journey. You are still that same girl, my love, in your spirit and your determination, in your smile and your laughter and in your humour and your being.

I see this so much now as Rosie progresses, marking her recovery in many ways. On her birthday, attending a Frank Turner gig in Exeter, standing cheek to jowl in the centre of the concert crowd, singing along to all the old stuff and the new. Happily making cupcakes in the kitchen while singing along to another favourite band, Bastille. Rosie has an amazing ability to keep herself upbeat, to pull herself out of the doldrums, even after these long years of difficult change.

We can still laugh at so many funny things, for instance finding a piece of freshly peeled ginger in the butter dish instead of butter, and odd things like that. She now picks me up on the things I forget and regularly empties my bath water when I forget to let it out and is so often one step ahead of me with her organisation.

Current thinking regarding the brain's ability to be more 'plastic' in its healing has helped us as a family to understand its potential. It has been the one thing that has enlightened and encouraged us more than anything, particularly now that we have had the experience of witnessing Rosie's recovery journey in the way we have.

The belief – held for years and years – that sustaining an acquired brain injury meant limitations to a person's life and to their potential has fortunately been rewritten. It gives hope where once there would have been none. Despite the life changes that often come with the injury, the potential for a brain to rewire and heal given the right conditions is so encouraging.

We still so often get the pitying looks and sighs from well-meaning folk when asked about Rosie's recovery and I have at times reached the point of doubting my own repeated, long-playing sentences. We have always remained positively beside her in her desire to return to London and regain her independence from us, but we have sometimes sensed that others, particularly those unwilling to change their perception of brain injury, are more sceptical. Many have perhaps thought we are in denial, having false hope or not facing up to our reality, especially as they observe Rosie still living at home and spending so long with us in Dorset, being held back as she is by the length of her court case. But we think differently.

Rosie is still making improvements in her executive functioning, the area of the brain responsible for planning and processing of information. This challenge so often hampers the daily lives of brain injury survivors and makes it difficult for them to carry out tasks consistently. Rosie had very good skills in this area before her accident so perhaps had a good starting point. She has been very conscientious in her daily programme of brain improvement exercises which I'm sure has helped her immensely. A great example of this functioning improving was when she recently made a cake. The tin she used was smaller than the size given in the recipe. I suggested the raw cake mixture would rise and overflow out of the tin and onto the oven floor during baking. Rosie, sharp as a knife, retorted, "The cake doesn't contain any raising agent so it's unlikely that would happen." My years of catering experience had just been trumped, big time.

The more we move on through these years of adjustment and improvement the more I realise just how fortunate we are to still have Rosie in our lives. I have just finished reading a book that has helped to confirm this to me so profoundly. It is *The Last Act of Love* by Cathy Rentzenbrink, a tender and beautifully composed book, written by the sister of a family having to make the desperate decision to end the life of her brother, his brain damage so profound that he would never get any better. He was knocked down by a car, too, his accident occurring in the year of Rosie's birth, twenty-something years ago. The circumstances of an accident, the time, the place and the century are so crucial to someone's survival and outcome. We have been granted the best of all three: the time of the morning when few other cars were on the road; the place, so close to a major hospital for the immediate and expert care Rosie received; the twenty-first century, modern medicine and research that increases the chances of survival after brain injury. I guess we got lucky.

Chapter 40

London: the Next Junction

Now that liability has been established in Rosie's court case – four and a half years since we began this long haul – we can at last feel confident that Rosie can move back into life again with the initial support to get her feet back on the ground and security for her future challenges. No one really wins in these difficult legal situations, as all the lives of those involved are affected to a greater or lesser degree. We still have a long way to go before the case is finally settled but, for now, we are just grateful that Rosie has been given some initial funding and can now start to prepare to embrace her independent life again.

This long period of time she has spent in Dorset that has been so critical to her brain and body healing is finally drawing to a close; she is so much stronger now. Time has helped her more than anything else. It has allowed her to come closer towards her own acceptance of her new self and she still needs more time to adjust as further acceptance will only come as she moves forward into her new life. Rosie's new challenges are acknowledged, and her differences are not deterring her or dampening her spirit. This feisty girl has got her fight still. She has yet to find her new niche in life and I am excited as to what her next calling will be. This next path she will tread could be quite something.

The hardest things can sometimes be the right things and this is all of that, my love. I know you are strong, but be wise and mindful as you tread your new road ahead; embrace this newness with your beautiful self, your zest, your vigour, your kindness. Open your heart and your mind to new horizons and new possibilities. Fill your broken parts with the golden joinery of an ancient Japanese vase; you will be more beautiful and more loved than ever before. The world is your oyster now, my darling girl, and this is your new beginning.

My feeling is "London nearly killed her – I hope London can now rebuild her." Our wonderful capital, there is a lot resting on you. Rosie has been given a second chance at life that's often denied to so many and, despite this challenging and changing world we live in, LIFE IS FOR LIVING, and that is just what she plans to do.

By the waters of the Thames,
I resolve to start again,

To wash my feet and cleanse my sins,
to lose my cobwebs on the wind,

To fix the parts of me I broke,
to speak out loud the things I know,

I haven't been myself.

'The Angel Islington' – Frank Turner

And for me? This curveball has made me realise just how fragile our lives are. Life is an ever-changing pattern; nothing stays the same as it shapes, moves and twists with each turn it takes: the good, the bad and sometimes the downright ugly. But this is all we have, and each day is a gift that is not granted to us all. This path has tested my unconditional love and my kindness and I have learnt that there are no bounds to the love you can have for your family when difficult times arrive at your doorstep, though this may not always be obvious until the tumult settles down.

Your children never stop teaching you things way into their adulthood; and the psychologist at Queen Mary's Hospital was right – I think you do, over time, appreciate life in a different way after tragedy. Our family has now moved to that point, I think, and we have learnt a lot from these last years.

I shall live each day with the gratitude that I still have my family and I have never touched wood on my bedside again since that November night. I know now that we are powerless to change what lies ahead of us, however much we worry and anguish over what the future holds.

I will take pleasure in the smallest of things and maybe, just maybe in the future I will return to my garden and grow vegetables again, now that my lovely family have cleared the thick matted brambles and the many years' worth of weeds. They long for me to pick up this important thread of my life again and I know in my heart that I yearn to see my garden thrive and feel the soil under my fingernails; it's so much part of my DNA.

It will go a long way to bridge this open gap, to heal the wounds and reunite me with this constant that I miss in my life. I want to feed my children all the goodness from my soil again when they visit, just like I used to... Somehow, though, I don't think I will be growing onions again any time soon...

Afterword:
Ten Years On – 2024

Ten years on ... I have to say these words out loud sometimes. There were many times when I could never have imagined life ten years on from 11th November 2014. Rosie has made so much progress since finally moving back to London in 2019. Funding from the insurance company has meant that she could have support, companionship, and a roof over her head. Rosie has taken up tennis, which has been a massive breakthrough in her recovery. Racquet sports offer so much in terms of our brains and physical body working together. She is now able to move freely around the court without thinking about where she places each foot. This, in turn, has really improved her memory. Sport has such a huge benefit to brain injury recovery. I really wish it could be more integrated within brain injury rehabilitation.

Rosie now lives independently, with support where she needs it. Her court case has finally been settled after all these years. A huge weight has been lifted from our shoulders.

As soon as the case settled, the driver of the car was finally given permission to reach out to us, the first opportunity since the day of the accident. Adrian and I agreed to a meeting in the hope of enabling some closure. It was an emotional few hours. We met a kind, honest and warm human who has carried a huge burden throughout these years. We were all able to put faces to the names that have been bandied around on legal papers for so long. To know that we don't blame and that we come from a human place, we hope, has eased some pain. To be open and honest with each other, a kind of reparative reconciliation, has been so beneficial to us all.

One day, Rosie may well meet the driver. For her, this accident changed her life so it will certainly be harder for her to process a potential meeting than it has been for us. She has not discounted it, and we feel sure it could be so helpful to both parties involved.

Sadly, dear old Monty has now passed away. This amazing dog had been unconditional in his therapy for Rosie. Over her recovery years at home, he had been her loving companion in so many ways. She Facetimed him to say goodbye and thanked him for helping her to walk again. These words reduced us all to tears.

Adrian and I are now happily retired in Dorset, spending our time pottering in our cottage and garden, surrounded by glorious countryside. I realise I am at my most contented when picking our home-grown vegetables for suppers and flowers to fill our cottage with beauty and pleasure. To have these simple constants that have kept me grounded throughout my life is pure joy. We count our blessings every day that Rosie is where she is, and we are where we are. Our lives could have turned out so differently. Gratitude is always and forever present in our lives. Our family continues its healing, with more beautiful grandchildren arriving and regular get-togethers. The power of family knows no bounds.

Rosie can finally move on to the next phase of her life and prove to herself what she is capable of achieving.

With a supportive partner now by her side, the sky is the limit. Obviously, she lives within her limitations and the constant effects of her injuries – memory fog and fatigue, to name a few – will be with her for her lifetime. To others, the only clue to her back story is her trachi scar. Behind that scar is her own story which is truly remarkable. This is my story. Rosie's is still waiting to be told...

~ The end ~

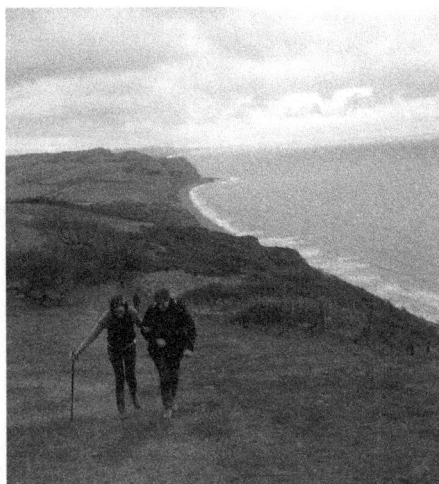

Walking to the top of Golden Cap:
11th November 2015.

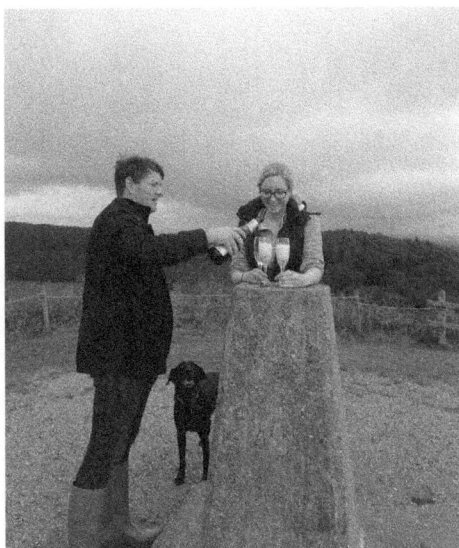

Celebrating at the top of Golden Cap – one year on!

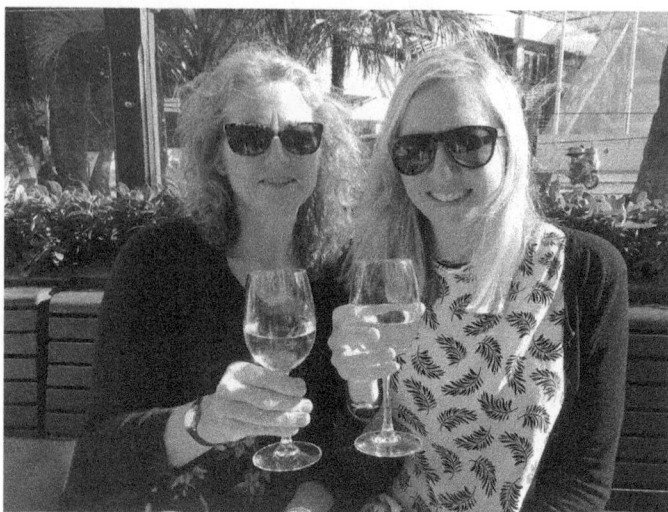

Celebrating in Nice – two years on.

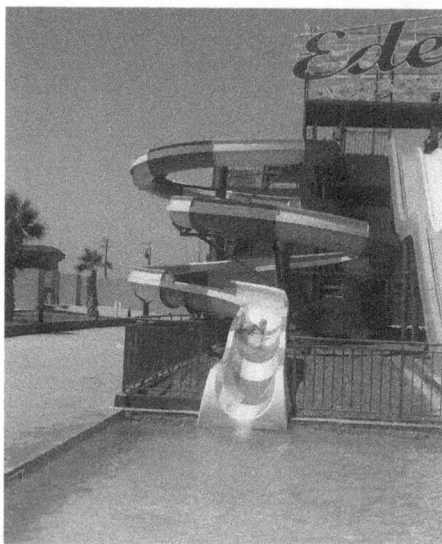

At the water park in Marrakesh: Summer 2017.

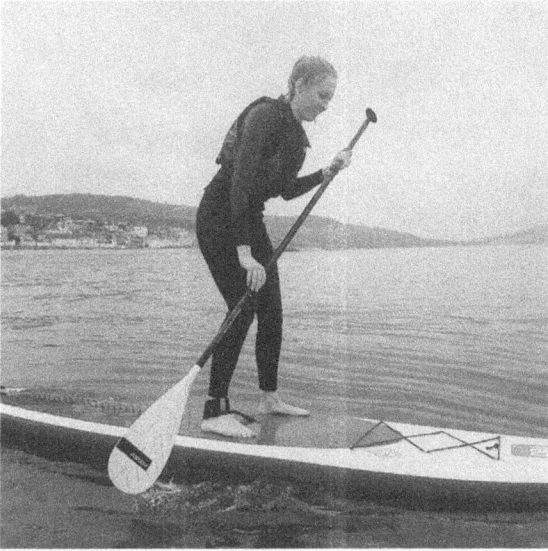

Paddleboarding in Lyme Bay: Summer 2018.

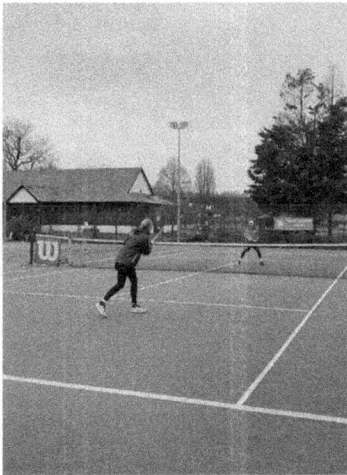

Playing tennis in Wimbledon: 2021.

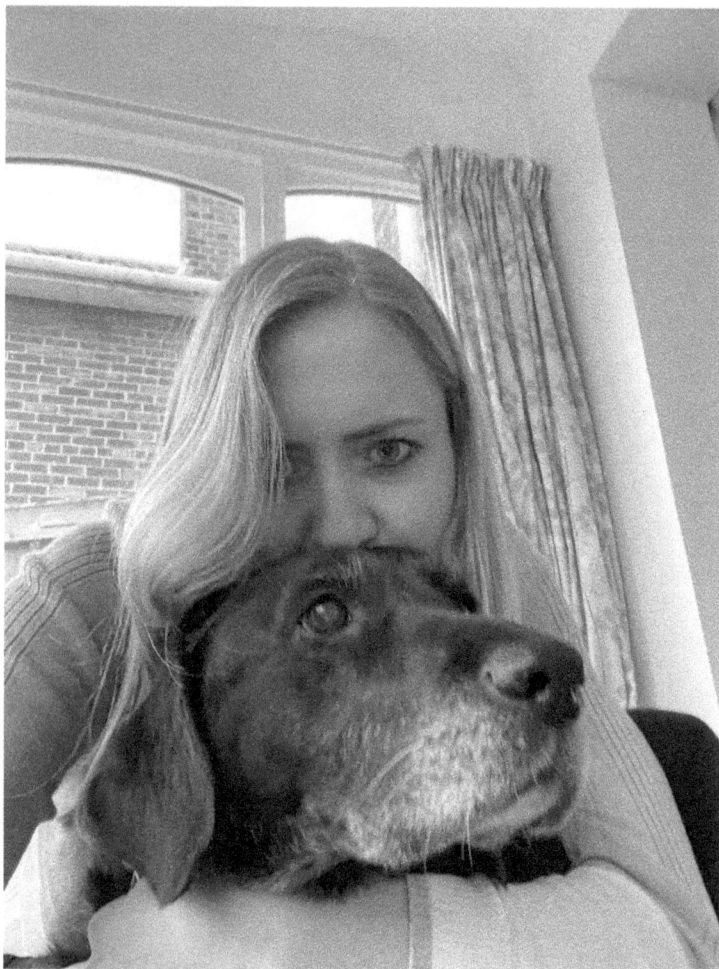

Rosie and Monty: 2022.

Author's Note

I have often doubted myself and my writing as I have no real grasp of English grammar and my spelling has always been suspect. I have tried hard not to let these issues discourage me from putting pen to paper for my book. I thoroughly recommend, whatever your standard of literacy, that you attempt to put your feelings down in words; you never know where it might lead, and the cathartic benefits are countless.

Little hints and tips to stay positive

1. Look after yourselves as well as your loved one – you are all in for the long haul so you may as well make life as comfortable as possible. By topping up your own engine tanks you will have the energy you need to support. Take regular exercise in fresh air; this helps to empty your head and fuel your energy levels.

2. It's hard not to feel guilty at times for doing this but it's vitally important that you don your comfortable clothes, switch off with some mindless telly, have some tasty food and a glass of something nice to help relax you at the end of these exhausting days. Maintain your old routines and habits, however small they are, to give you a sense of normality.

3. Get to know the hospital staff around you and up-skill yourself to understand what's going on. This can really help with reassurance and will make you

feel you are supported and not alone in what can be a very scary and daunting place.

4. Try, if possible, not to Google too much; it can really bring you to some very dark and often inaccurate conclusions. Let things evolve as they will inevitably do and cope with the here and now as much as possible.

5. Never lose sight of the character of your loved one who is suffering. Keep fighting, however hard this is at times, to bring out the best in them. Try not to make too many comparisons with the past and embrace and build on the new strengths they show.

6. Keep life on a light-hearted level as much as possible. Take note of the funny things that will inevitably lift your spirits up – laughter can so often be the best medicine of all.

7. Remember, every brain is different; Rosie is living proof of that. Recovery continues to take place for years to come, and that can make anything possible!

8. Life is a changing and movable feast; it will still go on regardless, so keep with it and accept things as they move along – it will get better.

9. Enjoy the simple things. Rosie has taught me that, in many ways. A slow walk is as replenishing as a fast brisk one; you can take the time to see the little things around you that sometimes get missed.

10. Enjoy as many things together as possible – each day is a day you could so easily not have been granted.

Glossary of Terms

CT scan – Computed tomography scan

EEG – Electroencephalogram

GCS – Glasgow Coma Scale

HEMS – Helicopter Emergency Medical Service

ICP – intracranial pressure bolt

ITU – Intensive Therapy Unit

Max fax – Maxillofacial

MDT – Multi Disciplinary Team

NG tube – Nasogastric tube

Physios – Highly specialised neuro-physiotherapists

PTA – Post Traumatic Amnesia

REM – Rapid Eye Movement

Trachi – Tracheotomy

Thanks and Acknowledgements

Our most sincere and grateful thanks go to the many amazing staff of St George's Hospital, Tooting, HEMS and the London Ambulance Service, and we are talking about hundreds of members of staff who saved Rosie's life and cared for her during her time in hospital. Their dedication, commitment and expertise are second to none; and now having had first-hand experience of NHS care from critical through to community care, we can honestly say it has been incredible in every sense. We will forever be in your debt.

To Dr Colette Griffin for kindly writing the foreword to my book and who gave us so much hope, keeping us on an 'even keel' during our hospital visits, and who continues to keep in touch with Rosie to this day.

To the Wolfson rehabilitation centre at St George's and Queen Mary's and both the Dorset and St John's Wandsworth Community Brain Injury teams who have helped and supported Rosie through her rehabilitation journey.

To the London Metropolitan Police Service, whose swift action helped save Rosie's life on the day of her accident.

To the gentleman who stayed by Rosie's side on the morning of her accident.

To Headway, the brain injury charity – for help and support particularly through their website which was, and still is, our reference tool in so many ways.

To Moore Barlow solicitors and Rosie's legal team for all their hard work to secure funding for the next stage of her life.

To 'Team Rosie' for continued rehabilitation support.

To Emma and Emma Wells Tennis team, Wimbledon for your amazing input.

To Coffee in the Wood, Colliers Wood and Tartan Artisanal, Tooting to name just two of the many coffee shops for their welcome, food and shelter on a regular basis.

Special thanks to Dani and Greg for your amazing support and for holding the family together on many occasions.

To Monty: you were a dog with a special gift and greatly loved by us all. RIP.

To Lauren, for your strength and resourcefulness; they are such admirable qualities.

To East Devon Health and Fitness and Lindsey, for making the difference to Rosie's physical recovery.

To Deborah Gildersleeves for being there for both Rosie and me.

To the Headspace meditation app and Andy, for keeping me in touch mentally.

To Sam Neal Yoga and Sam, for keeping me in touch physically.

To our Friends and Family and many others for all their support. You know who you are.

To Frank Turner, who has so very kindly permitted me to use his incredible lyrics in my book. Frank is one of Rosie's favourite artists; she could remember his song lyrics almost word for word during the early stages of her recovery.

To Weetabix – for being so kind in permitting me to use this word within my book.

To Fearne Cotton – whose familiar voice possibly stimulated Rosie to speak again.

To Cindy, my dear friend, for the first edit.

To Penny Dunscombe, for the final edit, whose expertise and painstaking attention to detail have transformed my pages of words into a proper book.

To Alastair, for turning my drawing into a front cover.

References and Copyright

Chapter 1

'Hope is the thing with feathers' – Emily Dickinson.

Chapters 1 and 5

Glasgow coma scale:
Glasgow coma scale.org/Wikipedia.org

Chapter 5

Westmead Post Traumatic Amnesia scale classification: Wikipedia.org

Diffuse Axonal Injury: Healthline.com/Wikipedia

Headway Brain Injury: www.headway.org.uk

Traumatic Brain Injury information manual: – St George's Healthcare NHS Trust

Chapter 11

A Tale for the Time Being – Ruth Ozeki, Canon Gate Books Ltd 2013

Chapter 12

My Stroke of Insight – Jill Bolte Taylor PhD - Hodder and Stoughton 2008

Chapter 29

Weetabix Ltd – who have sent me a letter confirming my use of the word 'Weetabix'

Chapter 32

Extract 'On Children' from *The Prophet* – Kahlil Gibran 1923 (Pan Books)

Chapter 39

The Last Act of Love – Cathy Rentzenbrink, Picador 2016

Introduction, Chs. 5, 21, 28, 39, 40

Song lyrics by Frank Turner, Artist and Musician – © and ® Xtra Mile Recordings published by BMI. Email confirmation of this approval.

www.ingramcontent.com/pod-product-compliance
Lightning Source LLC
Chambersburg PA
CBHW021616270326
41931CB00008B/717

*9 7 8 1 8 3 6 1 5 1 8 9 0 *